ANTI-INFLAMMATORY RECIPES

How to Reduce Inflammation in the Gut by Restoring Your Inner Balance

Artsy Chef

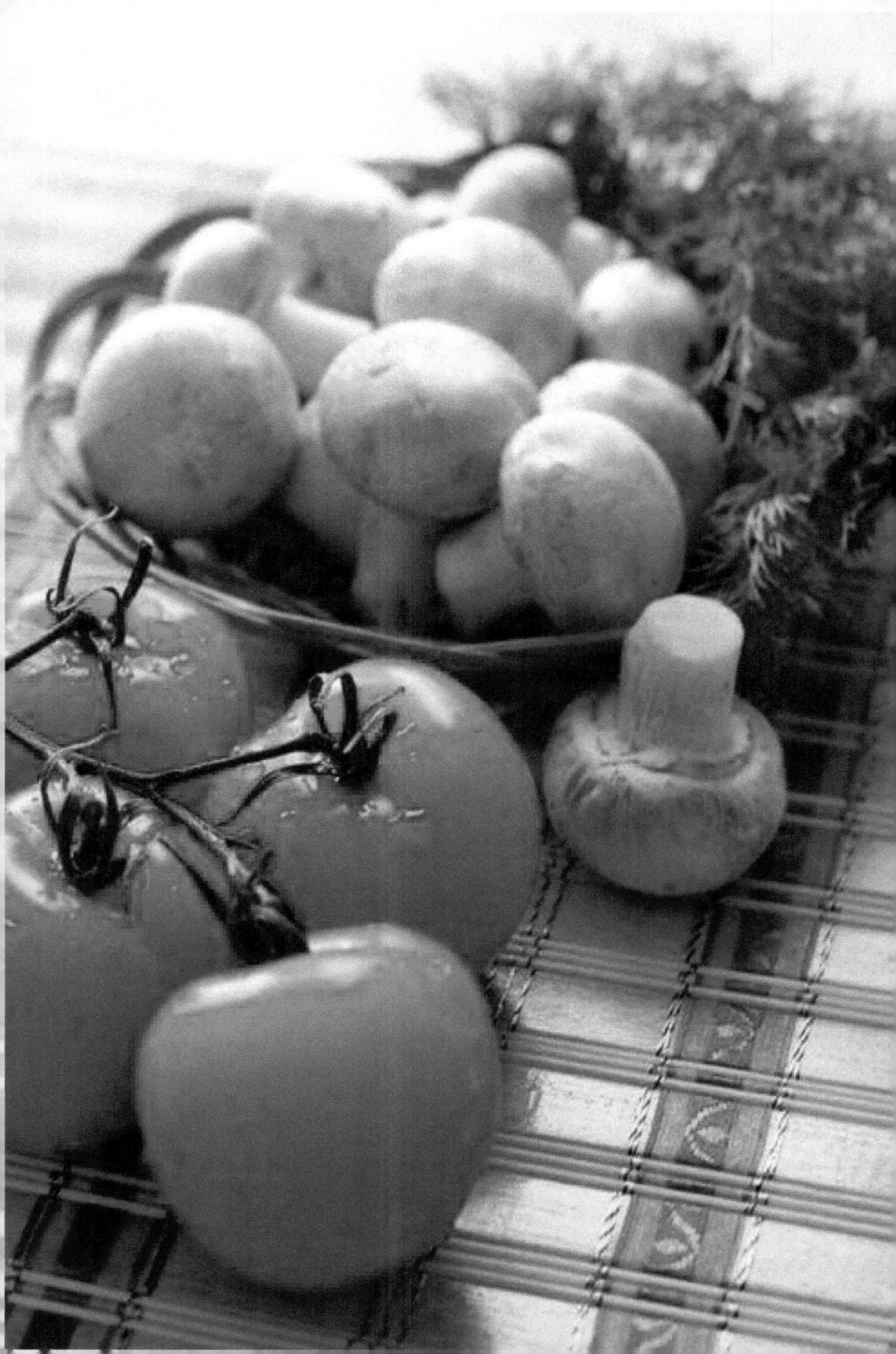

Table of Contents

INTRODUCTION

The anti-inflammatory diet is the best diet for conditions that cause inflammation such as asthma, chronic peptic ulcer, tuberculosis, rheumatoid arthritis, period on it is Crohn's disease, sinusitis, active hepatitis, etc. Along with medical treatment, proper nutrition is very important. An anti-inflammatory diet can help to reduce the pain from inflammation and supplement other treatments.

Inflammation is a natural response of your body to infections, injuries, and illnesses. The classic symptoms are redness, pain, heat, and swelling. Nevertheless, some diseases such as diabetes, heart disease, and cancer produce no symptoms. An anti-inflammatory diet is a great preventive way to safeguard your health.

The anti-inflammatory diet provides antioxidants and reduces the level of free radicals in our bodies. The most common question that people ask is what to eat while on the anti-inflammatory diet. Recommended foods are fruit, vegetables, whole grains, plant-based proteins, and fish, as well as spices, condiments, and dressings. The only condition that should be followed is that all food should be organic.

The most popular vegetables and fruits for the diet are leafy greens, cherries, raspberries, blackberries, tomatoes, cucumbers, etc. Grains include oatmeal, brown rice, and all grains that are high in fiber. Herbs and spices are natural antioxidants that will boost your health as they add flavor. You should avoid highly processed food such as sugary drinks, chocolate, ice cream, French fries, burgers, sausages, deli meats, and overly greasy food. One more factor that will help is making sure you get enough water per day. It is easy to track. There are a lot of apps that will help you to do it correctly. Drinking plenty of water helps the body to cleanse faster.

The anti-inflammatory diet is simple to follow and is not restrictive. There are many ways to adjust it to your preferences. Nevertheless, there are some cons that you should know. It can be costly since it recommends eating all organic food. It also contains a lot of allergens such as nuts, seeds, and soy.

However, eating the right adjusted food will help to eliminate the cons of the diet. It is highly recommended to go to your doctor for a complete medical examination before starting the diet.

This is important information that you should know before starting any diet. A diet is not a magic remedy for all diseases, but it does support the body in conjunction with treatment. Start your new healthy life with one small step, and you will see huge results within half a year. You can be sure that your body will respond by giving you a fresh look and energy for new achievements.

What to Eat and Avoid on the Anti-Inflammatory Diet

- **Meat, Poultry, and Fish**

The best choice for an anti-inflammatory diet is fish and seafood. This type of food is rich in omega-3 fatty acids. Meat can be eaten in moderation, although it is recommended to eat grass-fed meat.

What to eat	Eat occasionally	What to avoid
Tuna	Beef	Lamb
Sole	Chicken	Lard
Shrimps	Pork loin	Bacon
Turkey	Pork tenderloin	pork
Halibut		Breaded fish
Trout		
Salmon		
Flounder		

Mackerel		
Oysters		
Sardines		
Catfish		
Clams		
Cod		

- **Dairy**

Dairy products can be both useful and harmful to your health. Full-fat dairy products can cause acne and increase inflammatory conditions.

What to eat	Eat occasionally	What to avoid
Non-fat milk	Rice milk	Whole cream
Low-fat milk	Skim milk	Sour cream
Coconut milk	Tofu cheese	Cream
Greek-style	Parmesan	Hard cheese

yogurt		Milk butter
Fat-free plain traditional yogurt		Margarine
		Cottage cheese
Cashew butter		
Sunflower seeds butter		

- **Eggs**

Eggs contain essential nutrients, proteins, lutein, and zeaxanthin, which all fight inflammation. Nevertheless, frequent consumption of eggs can cause allergic reactions.

- **Nuts and Seeds**

Nuts and seeds are good for heart health. They are rich in fiber and nutrition. Only eat them if you're sure you have no sensitivities.

What to eat	Eat occasionally	What to avoid
Almonds	Hazelnuts	Chocolate-covered nuts
Chia seeds	Cashews	
Flaxseeds	Peanut butter	Nut butter (sweetened/ unsweetened)
Pumpkin seeds		Macadamia nuts
Pistachios		Peanuts
		Pecans

Vegetables

The main source of vitamins during the anti-inflammatory diet is vegetables. However, not all vegetables are beneficial. Avoid starchy vegetables and vegetables that can cause allergic reactions.

What to eat	Eat occasionally	What to avoid
Sweet potatoes	Tomatoes	Potatoes
Yams	Tomatillos	Potato chips
Beets	Corn	Mushrooms
Radishes		
Watermelon		
Green beans		
Organic baked corn chips		
Sweet peppers		
Shiitake mushrooms		
Bell peppers		

- **Fruits and Berries**

Fruits are rich in vitamins. Nevertheless, avoid eating large amounts of sugary fruits. Replace them with sweet and sour or sour fruits/berries.

What to eat	Eat occasionally	What to avoid
Tart cherries	Kiwi	Acerola
Strawberries	Papaya	Lychee
Blueberries	Bananas	Persimmon
Apples		
Pears		
Apricots		
Avocado		
Dried fruits		
Oranges		

Mangoes Pineapple		

- **Grain Products**

Whole-grains are rich in fiber and can fight inflammation and protect our body from infection. Avoid eating "bad" grains.

What to eat	What to avoid
Brown rice	White rice
Wild rice	Sugar cereals
Oatmeal	White bread
Whole-grain bread	Crackers
Multigrain bread	Snacks
Whole-grain pasta	Rye bread
Oat flour	Wheat noodles
Buckwheat flour	White bread crumbs
Whole wheat flour	Corn flour
Rice noodles	Wheat tortillas

| Corn tortillas | Bagels |
| Whole-grain toast | |

- **Condiments**

Condiments play a significant role in flavor. They can make a meal tender, spicy, or salty. On your anti-inflammatory diet, you can use almost all spices and herbs. They have strong anti-inflammatory features.

What to eat	What to avoid
Low-fat mayonnaise	Mayonnaise (full-fat)
Ground pink peppercorns	Tartar sauce
Turmeric tahini dressing	Teriyaki
Alfredo sauce	Tomato sauce
Hot red pepper sauce	Bordelaise sauce
Chimichurri sauce	Brown sauce
Curry powder	Chili sauce
Tapatio sauce (handmade)	Dijon sauce
Apple cider vinegar	Buffalo sauce
	Hollandaise sauce

Pomegranate sauce	Marinara sauce
	Worcestershire sauce
	Sweet and sour sauce
	Soy sauce
	Pickle relish
	Barbecue sauce
	Dijon mustard

- **Oils and fats**

It is recommended to consume vegetable oils and fats during the anti-inflammatory diet. Bear in mind that some natural oils can cause allergies.

What to eat	Eat occasionally	What to avoid
Sunflower oil (cold-pressed) Grapes seed oil	Walnut oil	Coconut oil Palm oil

Olive oil (extra virgin) Flax seeds oil		

- **Beverages**

Drinking water should be a rule for you during the anti-inflammatory diet. Nevertheless, not all drinks are created equal. Avoid consuming sparkling drinks and beverages that contain artificial sugars.

What to eat	Eat occasionally	What to avoid
Fresh fruits Seltzer Filtered water Mineral water Lemon water Herbal tea	Fresh juice	Coffee Sodas Wine Sparkling mineral water Carbonated drinks Sweet sparkling beverages

Green tea Mate tea		

- **Sweets**

Fruits are the best sweets during the anti-inflammatory diet. They are rich in vitamins and contain only natural sweeteners.

Nevertheless, you can find a lot of sugar-free meals which are not inferior in taste to the most famous desserts.

What to eat	Eat occasionally	What to avoid
Honey Raw cocoa powder Fruits (allowed for anti-inflammatory diet)	Stevia Xylitol Brown rice syrup Dark chocolate	Artificial sweeteners Buns Candy Cakes Chocolate Cookies

		Custard
		Ice cream
		Pastries
		Pies
		Pudding
		Sugar
		Tarts
		Corn syrup
		Milk chocolate

- **Beans and Legumes**

Consumption of beans and legumes is very important during the anti-inflammatory diet. They are rich in fiber and contain large amounts of protein as well as antioxidants. It is necessary to eat at least two servings of beans or legumes per week.

Note that beans and legumes can cause inflammation only if they are cooked in the wrong way. It is recommended to soak beans before cooking.

- **Others**

Fast food and processed food are forbidden during the anti-inflammatory diet. Such food damages our digestive and immune system.

Top 10 Anti-Inflammatory Diet Tips

- **Avoid white food**

Avoiding white food such as sugar, salt, etc. can help to maintain and control the normal level of blood sugar. Try to add more lean proteins and high fiber food to your daily diet. It can be lean types of meat, brown rice, and whole grains.

- **An apple a day keeps the doctors away**

Add vegetables, fruits, nuts, and spices to your daily meal plan. Garlic, ginger, cinnamon, and lemon will help to boost your immune system and reduce inflammation.

- **Exercise daily**

Regular sports activities can help to prevent inflammation. Do 5-10 minutes of exercise daily to feel healthier.

- **Balance your mind**

Everyday stress leads to chronic diseases. Practicing yoga, meditation, or biofeedback are excellent ways to balance your mind and manage stress.

- **Choose the right proteins**

Lean red meat can be served as a source of proteins but it is still high in cholesterol and salt. Instead, choose fish such as halibut, salmon, tuna, cod, or seabass. They are rich in omega-3 fatty acids.

- **Drink antioxidant beverages**

Herbs are a great source of antioxidants and promote faster treatment. Basil, thyme, oregano, chili pepper, and curcumin have high anti-inflammatory features and serve as natural painkillers.

- **Get enough sleep**

You should always get 8-9 hours of sleep at night. Too much or too little sleep is the main triggers for heart disease and type 2 diabetes.

- **Cross out alcohol from your diet**

Avoiding alcohol helps keep you calm and reduces the risk of inflammation.

Choose green tea instead of coffee or black tea.

Green tea can fight free radical damage. Drinking green tea regularly lowers the risk of cancer and Alzheimer's disease.

- **Consume probiotics every day**

Urban lifestyle and junk food is bad for your digestion. Eating food that is rich in probiotics like sauerkraut, yogurt, milk, kombucha, miso, kimchi, and fermented vegetables/fruits every day will improve your gut's microbe barrier.

BREAKFAST

Cucumber and Avocado Salad

6 Servings

Preparation Time: 10 minutes

Ingredients

- 1 pound cucumbers, chopped
- 2 tablespoons Olive oil
- 2 tablespoons lemon juice
- ¼ cup chopped Parsley
- A pinch of salt and black pepper
- 2 Avocados, pitted and chopped
- 1 small red Onion, thinly sliced

Directions

- In a mixing bowl, mix together the cucumbers with the avocados, onion, oil, lemon juice, parsley, salt and pepper.
- Serve for breakfast.

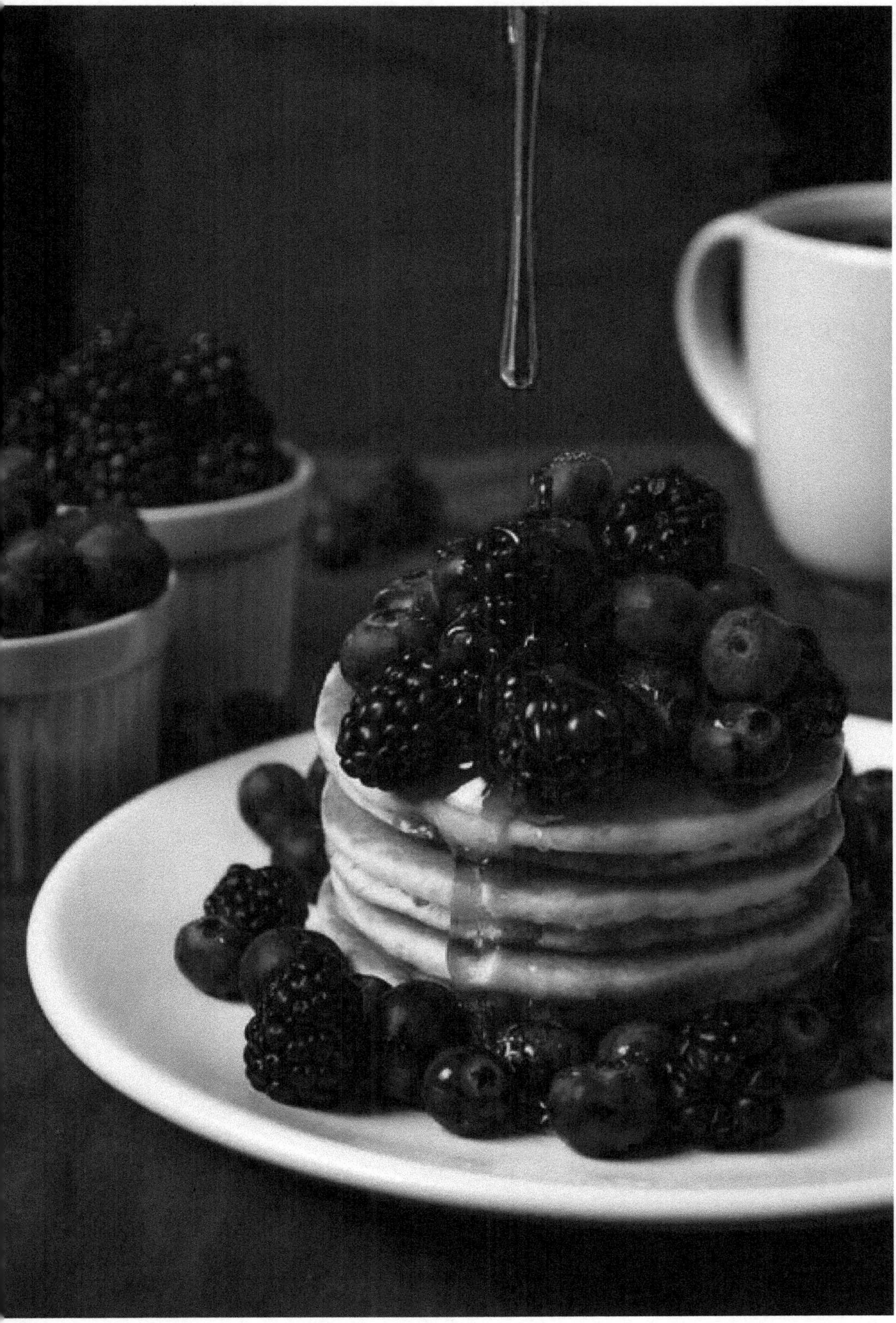

Watermelon Salad with Jalapeno

4 Servings

Preparation Time: 10 minutes

Ingredients

- ½ teaspoon Agave nectar
- 2 cups baby Arugula
- 2 tablespoons lemon juice
- 1 tablespoon extra-virgin Olive oil
- 1 Jalapeno, seeded and chopped
- 12 ounces Watermelon, chopped
- 1 red Onion, thinly sliced
- ½ cup chopped Basil leaves

Directions

- Take a bowl, toss together the Watermelon with the jalapeno, onion, basil, Arugula, oil, agave nectar, lemon juice and oil.
- Serve for breakfast.

Avocado Pork Tenderloin

6 Servings

Preparation Time: 10 minute

Ingredients

- 1-pound pork Tenderloin
- 1 tablespoon minced Garlic
- ¼ cup of Water
- ½ teaspoon Cayenne pepper
- 2 tablespoons Avocado oil

Directions

- Pour water into the baking pan.
- Then rub the pork tenderloin with avocado oil, minced garlic, and cayenne pepper.
- Add the meat into the pan with water and bake at 375° for 1 hour.

Fruit Bowl

4 Servings

Preparation Time: 10 minutes

Ingredients

- 2 Oranges, peeled, chopped
- 1 teaspoon Poppy seeds
- 1 tablespoon Coconut cream
- 1 teaspoon Coconut shred
- 1 Banana, chopped
- 2 Kiwis, peeled, chopped

Directions

- Mix oranges with a Banana in a mixing bowl.
- Add kiwis, poppy seeds, and Coconut shred. Gently shake the mixture.
- Top the meal with Coconut cream.

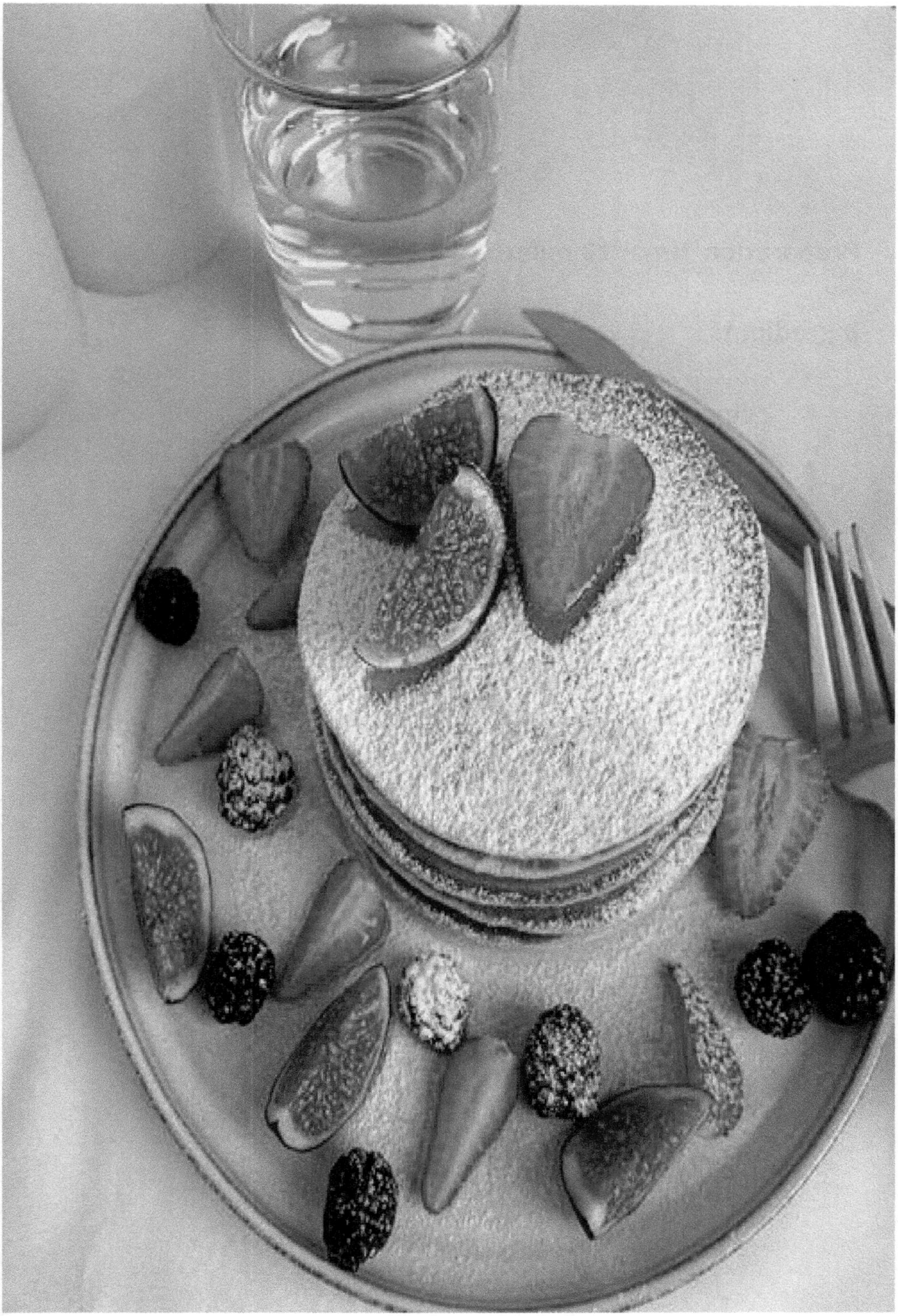

Vanilla Pudding

5 Servings

Preparation Time: 10 minutes

Ingredients

- 2 cups plain Yogurt
- ½ cup Strawberries, sliced
- 1 teaspoon Vanilla extract
- 4 tablespoons Chia seeds, dried

Directions

- Mix plain Yogurt with vanilla extract and chia seeds and leave for 15 minutes.
- Then transfer the pudding in the serving glasses and top with strawberries.

Ginger Pork Loins

6 Servings

Preparation Time: 50 minutes

Ingredients

- 4 pork Loins (3 oz each pork loin)
- 1 tablespoon Olive oil
- 1 teaspoon Lemon juice
- ¼ cup of Water
- 1 teaspoon minced ginger
- ½ teaspoon ground Ginger

Directions

- Rub the pork loins with minced Ginger, ground Ginger, Olive oil, and lemon juice.
- Then add the pork loins in casserole mold.
- Add water and cover the mold with foil.
- Bake the pork loins at 375° for 40 minutes.

Cashew Porridge

4 Servings

Preparation Time: 10 minutes

Ingredients

- 1 cup Cashew milk, warm
- 1 cup Apricots, chopped
- ½ cup Quinoa, cooked
- ¼ cup Pistachios, chopped
- 2 teaspoons raw Honey

Directions

- Mix quinoa with cashew milk.
- Transfer the mixture into the serving bowls.
- Top the quinoa with apricots, pistachios, and raw honey.

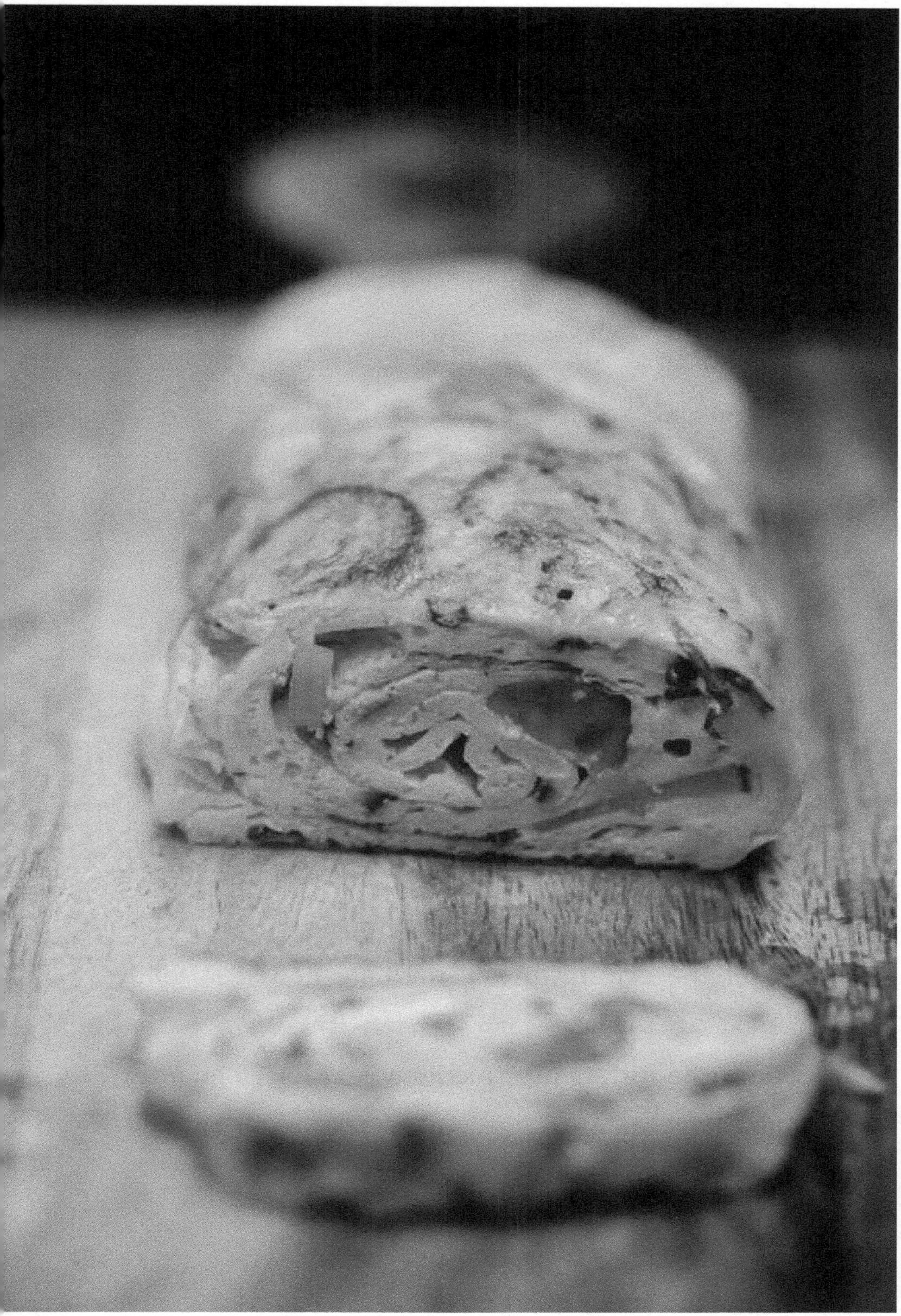

Parsley Frittata

6 Servings

Preparation Time: 30 minutes

Ingredients

- ¼ cup plain Yogurt
- ½ cup Parsley, chopped
- 1 teaspoon Olive oil
- ½ teaspoon Cayenne pepper
- 6 Eggs, beaten

Directions

- Mix plain Yogurt with eggs, parsley, and cayenne pepper.
- Then pour the Olive oil in the pan and preheat it well.
- Pour the egg mixture in the pan, flatten it gently and close the lid.
- Cook the frittata over medium heat for 20 minutes, and serve.

LUNCH

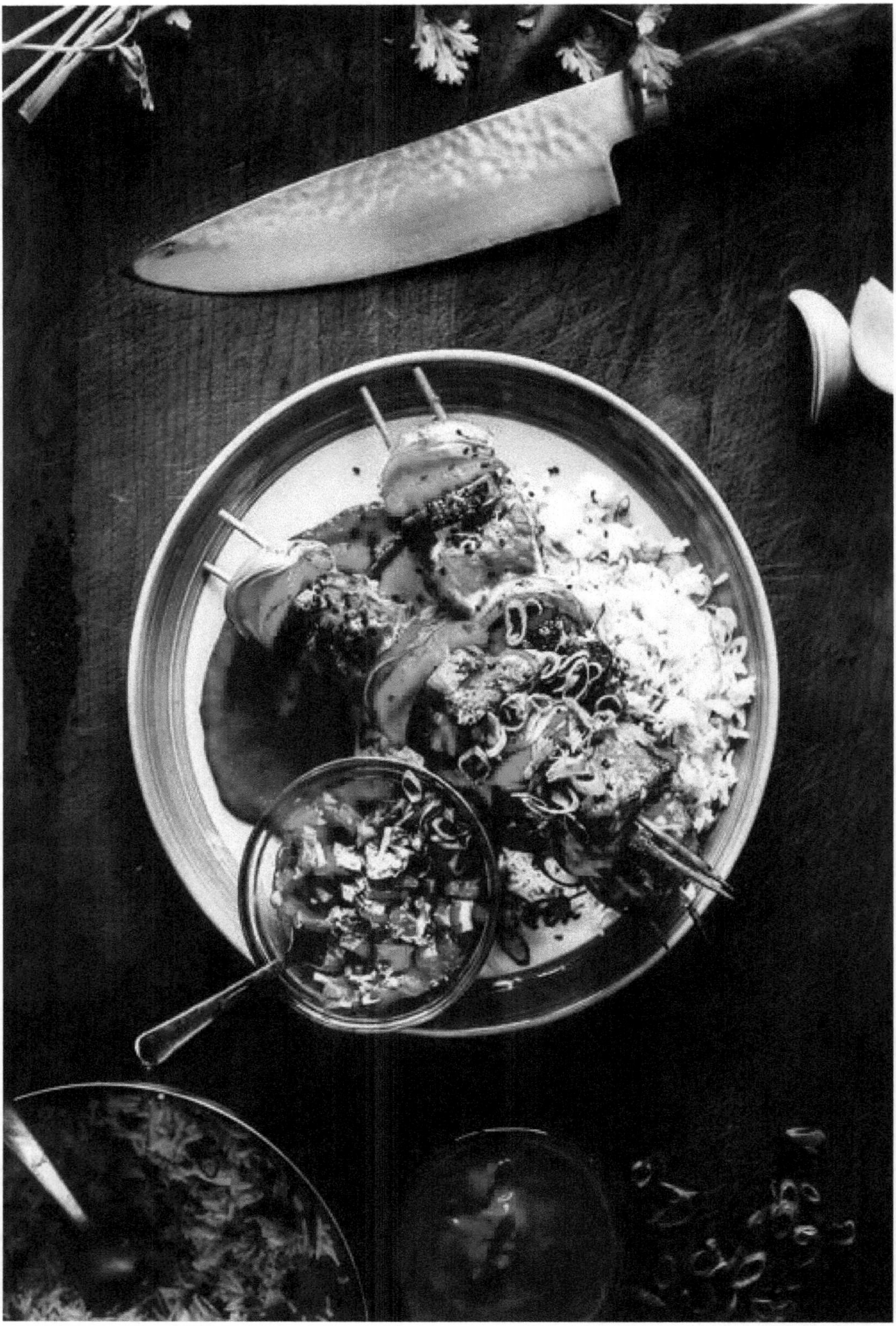

Baked Leek

6 Servings

Preparation Time: 30 minutes

Ingredients

- 1-pound leek, sliced
- 1 carrot, grated
- 1 cup of Coconut milk
- 1 teaspoon Olive oil
- 1 teaspoon ground black pepper

Directions

- Mix leek with grated carrot, Olive oil, ground black pepper, and Coconut milk.
- Add the mixture in the baking pan and flatten it gently.
- Bake the meal at 360° for 20 minutes.

Broccoli Steaks

5 Servings

Preparation Time: 30 minutes

Ingredients

- 1-pound broccoli head
- 1 teaspoon cayenne pepper
- 2 tablespoons Olive oil

Directions

- Slice the broccoli head into the steaks and Add in the baking tray in one layer.
- Sprinkle the vegetables with cayenne pepper and Olive oil.
- Bake the broccoli steaks at 365° for 10 minutes per side.

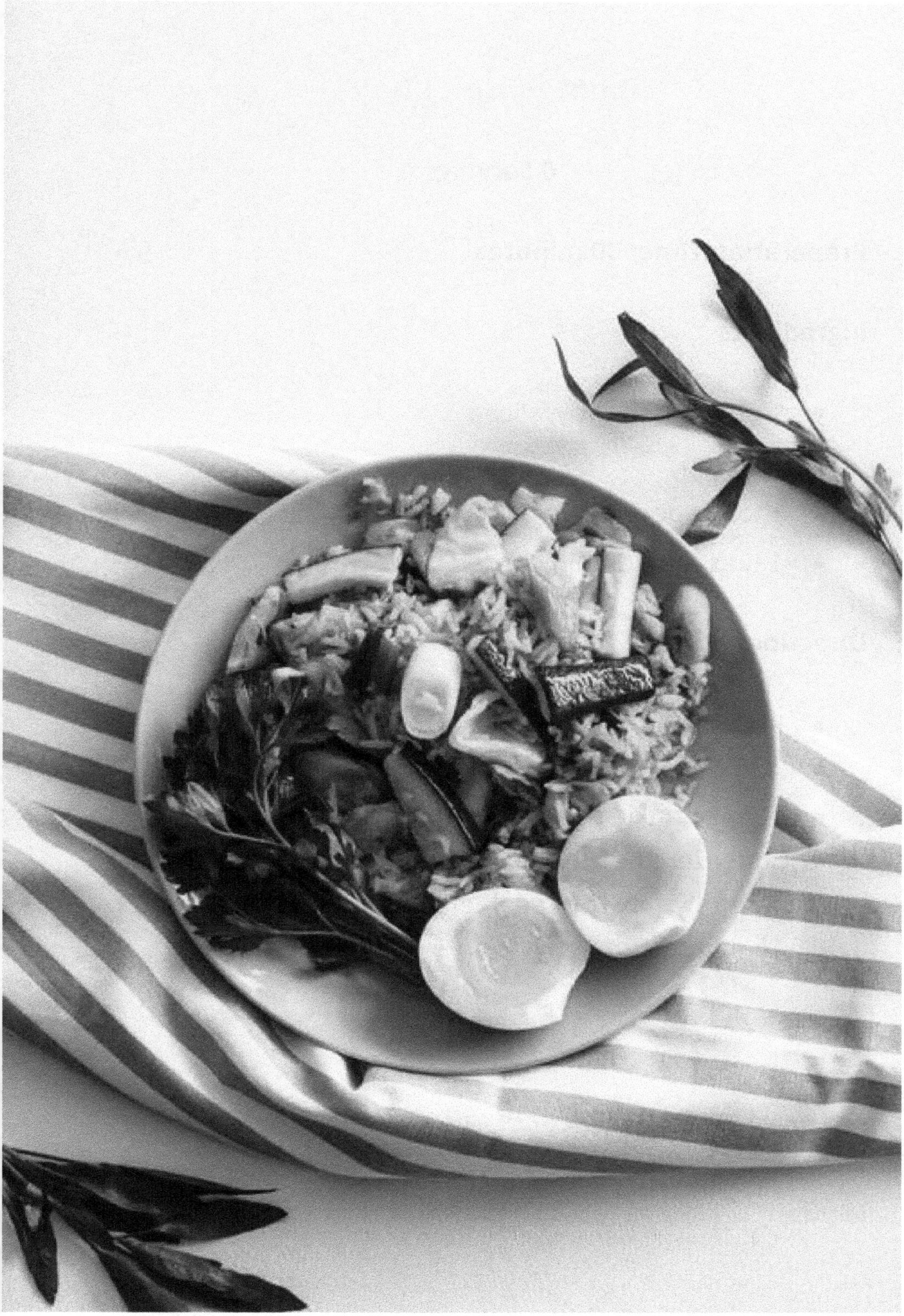

Lemon Bok Choy

6 Servings

Preparation Time: 30 minutes

Ingredients

- 1 pound bok choy, sliced
- 1 lemon
- 1 tablespoon Olive oil
- 1 teaspoon Cumin seeds

Directions

- Preheat the Olive oil in the pan well.
- Add bok choy and roast it for 1 minute per side.
- Then sprinkle the bok choy with cumin seeds.
- Squeeze the lemon juice over the bok choy, carefully mix the meal, and cook it on low heat for 15 minutes.

Parmesan Kale

6 Servings

Preparation Time: 25 minutes

Ingredients

- 4 cups kale, roughly chopped
- 2 oz Parmesan, grated
- 1 tablespoon Olive oil

Directions

- Add the kale in the tray and flatten it well.
- Then sprinkle the kale with Olive oil and Parmesan.
- Cook the kale at 350° for 20 minutes.

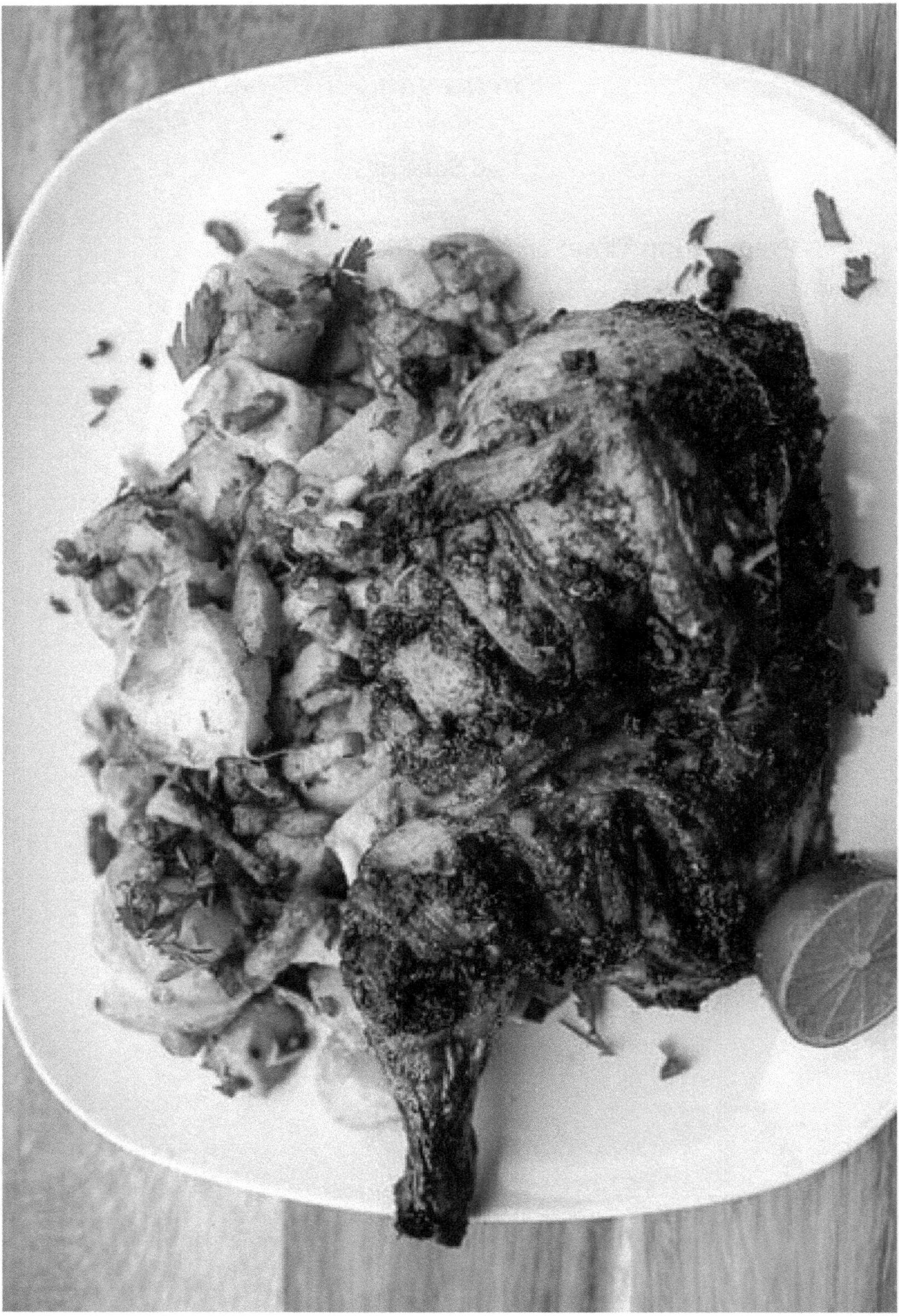

Curry Tofu

6 Servings

Preparation Time: 25 minutes

Ingredients

- 1-pound tofu, cubed
- 1 teaspoon curry powder
- 1 tablespoon Olive oil
- ½ cup Coconut cream
- 1 teaspoon lemon zest, grated

Directions

- In the mixing bowl, mix curry powder with Olive oil, Coconut cream, and lemon zest.
- Then add tofu and mix well.
- Leave the mixture for 10 minutes to marinate.
- Then preheat the pan well.
- Add tofu and cook it for 2 minutes per side.

Chickpeas Spread

2 Servings

Preparation Time: 10 minutes

Ingredients

- 1 cup chickpeas, cooked
- 1 tablespoon tahini paste
- 2 tablespoons lemon juice
- ¼ cup Olive oil

Directions

- Add all ingredients in the food processor.
- Blend the mixture until smooth.
- Transfer it in the serving bowl.

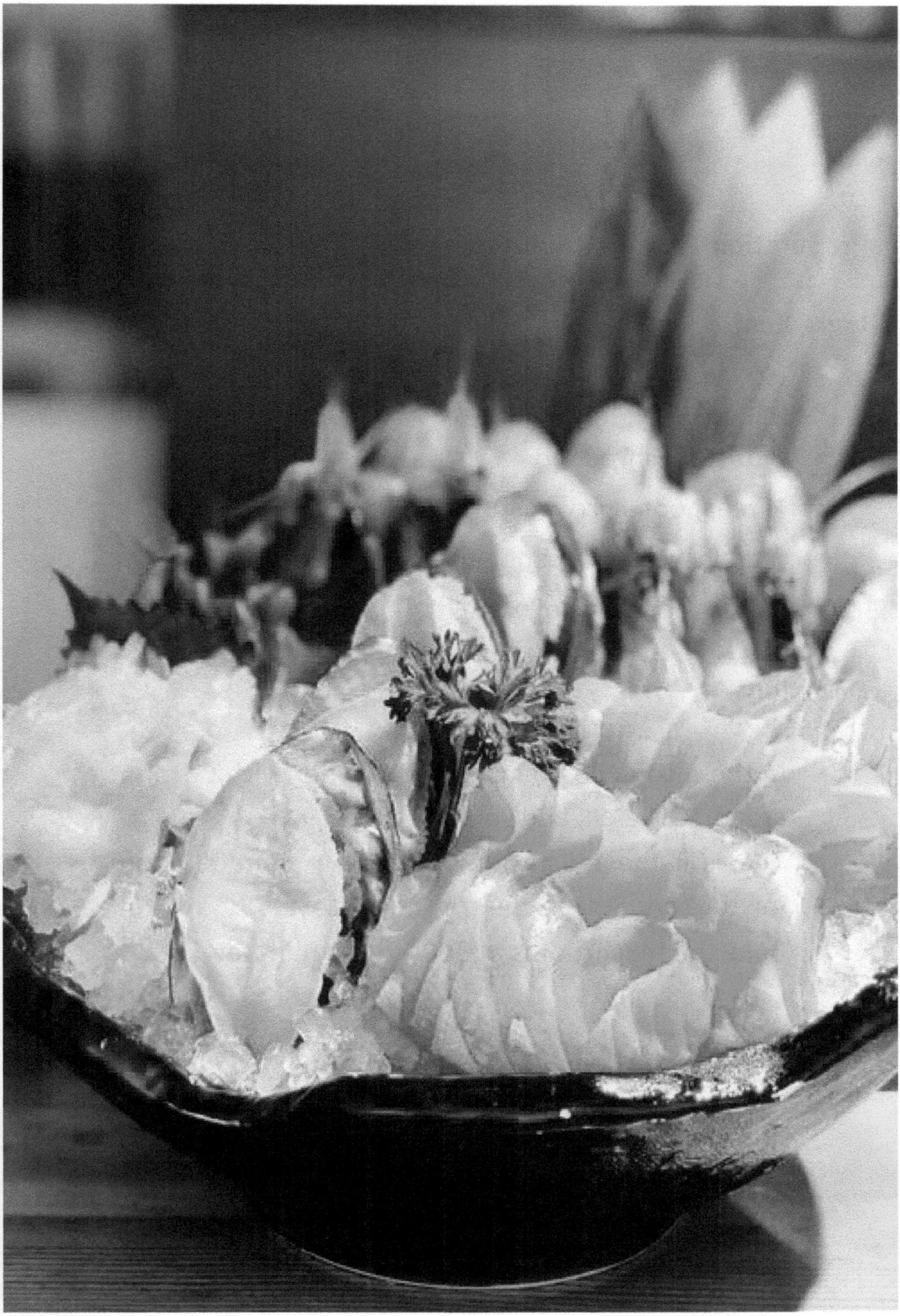

Mushroom Caps

6 Servings

Preparation Time: 30 minutes

Ingredients

- 5 Portobello Mushrooms(caps)
- 3 oz tofu, shredded
- ½ teaspoon curry paste
- 2 tablespoons Coconut cream
- 1 teaspoon Olive oil

Directions

- In the mixing bowl, mix curry powder with Coconut cream, Olive oil, and shredded tofu.
- Then fill the mushrooms with the shredded tofu mixture and Add in the tray in one layer.
- Bake the mushrooms at 360° for 20 minutes.

Ginger Baked Mango

6 Servings

Preparation Time: 30 minutes

Ingredients

- 2 mangos, pitted, halved
- 1 teaspoon minced Ginger
- 1 tablespoon Olive oil
- ¼ teaspoon dried rosemary

Directions

- Add the mango halves in the baking tray and sprinkle with Olive oil.
- Then sprinkle the fruit with minced ginger and dried rosemary.
- Bake the mango at 360° for 20 minutes.

SNACKS & APPETIZERS

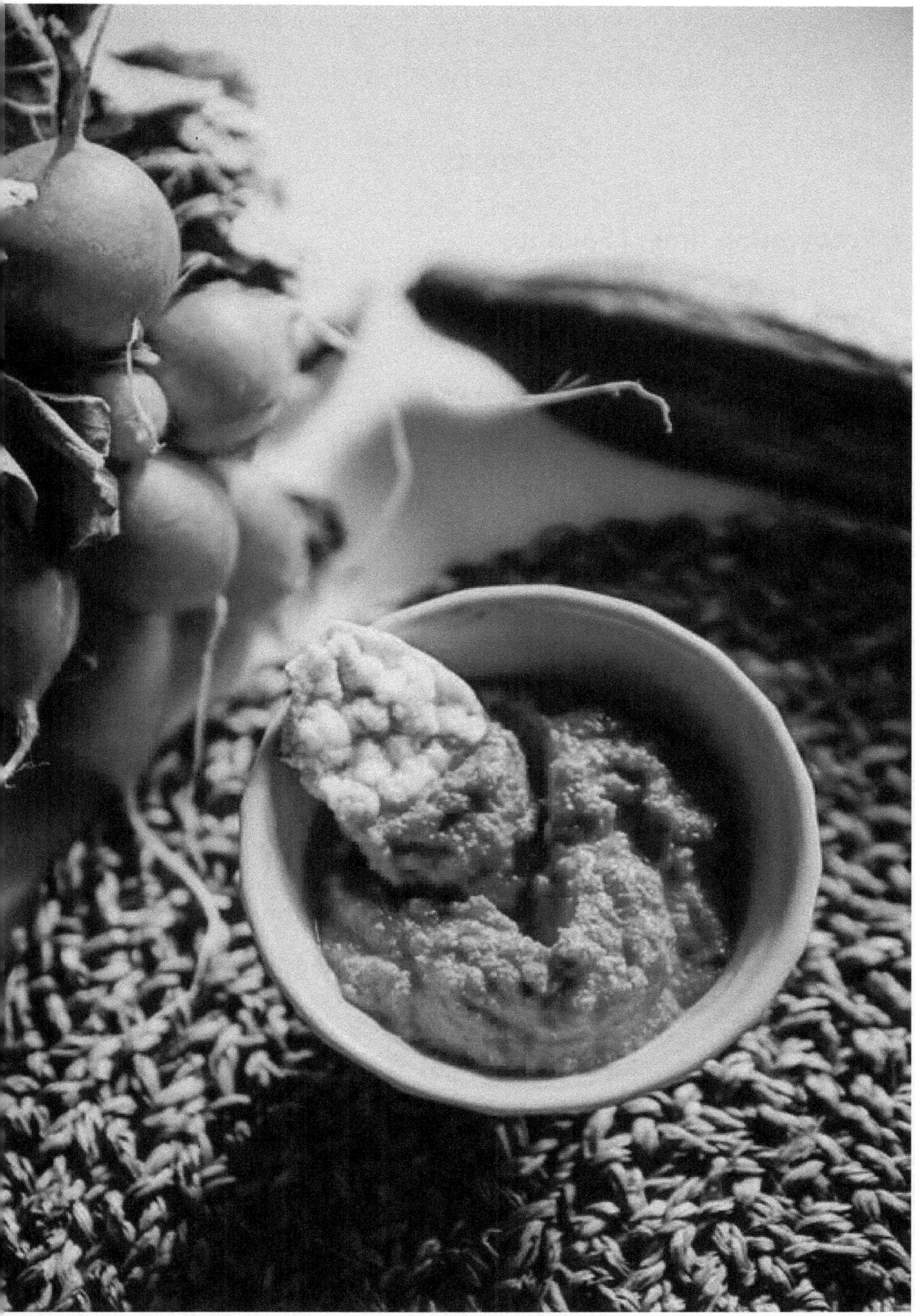

Seafood Appetizer Bowls

4 Servings

Preparation time: 25minutes

Ingredients

- 1 teaspoon Tomato paste
- 1 tablespoon Mayonnaise
- 1 teaspoon Lemon juice
- Salt and Black pepper to the taste
- ½ teaspoon ground Turmeric
- 8 ounces Calamari, cut into medium rings
- 7 ounces Shrimp, peeled and deveined
- 1 tablespoon Coconut oil, melted
- 2 tablespoons Avocado, chopped

Directions

- Grease a baking dish with the coconut oil; add calamari, shrimp, tomato paste, lemon juice, salt, pepper and turmeric.
- Toss and bake in the oven at 400°F for 15 minutes.
- Remove from the oven, add the avocado, toss and divide into bowls and serve as an appetizer.

Octopus with Celery Appetizer

4 Servings

Preparation time: 50minutes

Ingredients

- 3 ounces Olive oil
- Salt and Black pepper to the taste
- 4 tablespoons chopped Parsley
- 21-ounces Octopus, rinsed
- Juice of 1 Lemon
- 4 Celery stalks, chopped

Directions

- Put the octopus in a pot, add the water to cover, then cover the pot.
- Bring to a boil over medium heat and cook for 40 minutes.
- Drain, cool down the cooked octopus, chop and put in a salad bowl.

- Add the celery stalks, parsley, oil, salt, pepper and lemon juice.
- Mix it well, divide it into small bowls and serve as an appetizer.

Coconut Cream Clams Mix

6 Servings

Preparation time: 2 hours 10 minutes

Ingredients

- 2 cups Vegetable stock

- A drizzle of Olive oil

- 14 ounces canned Baby clams

- 2 cups Coconut cream

- 1 cup chopped Onion

- 1 cup chopped Celery stalks

- Salt and Black pepper to the taste

- 1 teaspoon Ground thyme

Directions

- Heat up a pan with the oil over medium heat and add the celery and onion. Stir and cook for 5 minutes.

- Transfer this mix to a Crockpot and add the baby clams, salt, pepper, stock, thyme and cream.
- Stir and cook on High for 2 hours, then divide into bowls and serve as an appetizer.

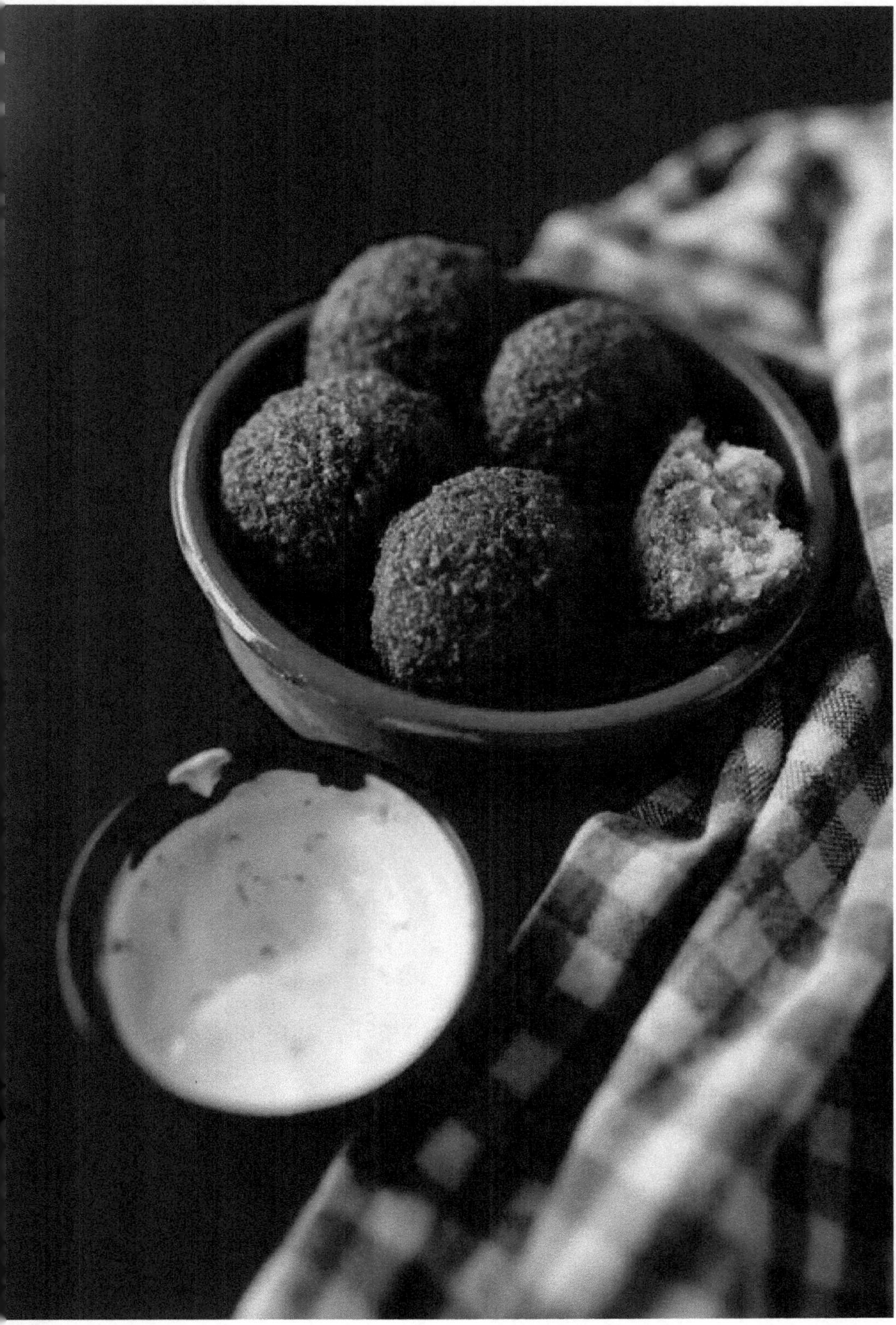

Endive with Herbed Shrimp Salad

6 Servings

Preparation time: 20minutes

Ingredients

- 3 tablespoons chopped Parsley
- 2 teaspoons chopped Mint
- 1 tablespoon chopped Tarragon
- 2 tablespoons Mayonnaise
- 1 teaspoon Lime zest
- 2 tablespoons Olive oil
- 1 pound Shrimp, peeled and deveined
- Salt and Black pepper to the taste
- 2 tablespoons Lime juice
- 3 Endives, shredded

Directions

- In a bowl, mix shrimp with salt, pepper and the olive oil.

- Toss to coat, then spread the shrimp on a lined baking sheet. Bake in the oven at 400°F for 10 minutes.
- Remove from oven and then add lime juice, toss and transfer to a bowl.
- Add the endive, parsley, mint, tarragon, mayo, and lemon zest.
- Toss it together and serve as an appetizer.

Citrus Oyster Platter

6 Servings

Preparation time: 10 minutes

Ingredients

- 1 Serrano Chili pepper, chopped
- 1 cup Tomato juice
- ½ teaspoon fresh grated ginger
- ¼ teaspoon minced garlic
- A pinch of Salt and Black pepper
- ¼ cup Olive oil
- ¼ cup chopped Cilantro
- ¼ cup chopped Scallions
- 12 Oysters, shucked
- Juice of 1 Lemon
- Juice of 1 Orange
- Zest of 1 Orange
- Juice of 1 Lime
- Zest of 1 Lime

Directions

- In a bowl, mix the lemon and the orange juice with lime zest, lime juice, orange zest, chili pepper, tomato juice, ginger, garlic, salt, pepper, oil, scallions and cilantro.
- Stir really well, then spoon this mixture into the oysters and serve them as an appetizer.

Salmon and Avocado Wraps

8 Servings

Preparation time: 10 minutes

Ingredients

- 6 ounces smoked Salmon, sliced

- 4 ounces Coconut cream

- 1 Cucumber, sliced

- 1 teaspoon Wasabi paste

- 2 Nori sheets

- 1 small Avocado, pitted, peeled and chopped

Directions

- Place the nori sheets on a sushi mat.
- Divide the salmon slices, avocado and cucumber slices on each piece of nori. In a bowl, mix together coconut cream with wasabi paste.

- Spread this over the cucumber and roll your nori sheets.
- Cut each into medium pieces and serve as an appetizer.

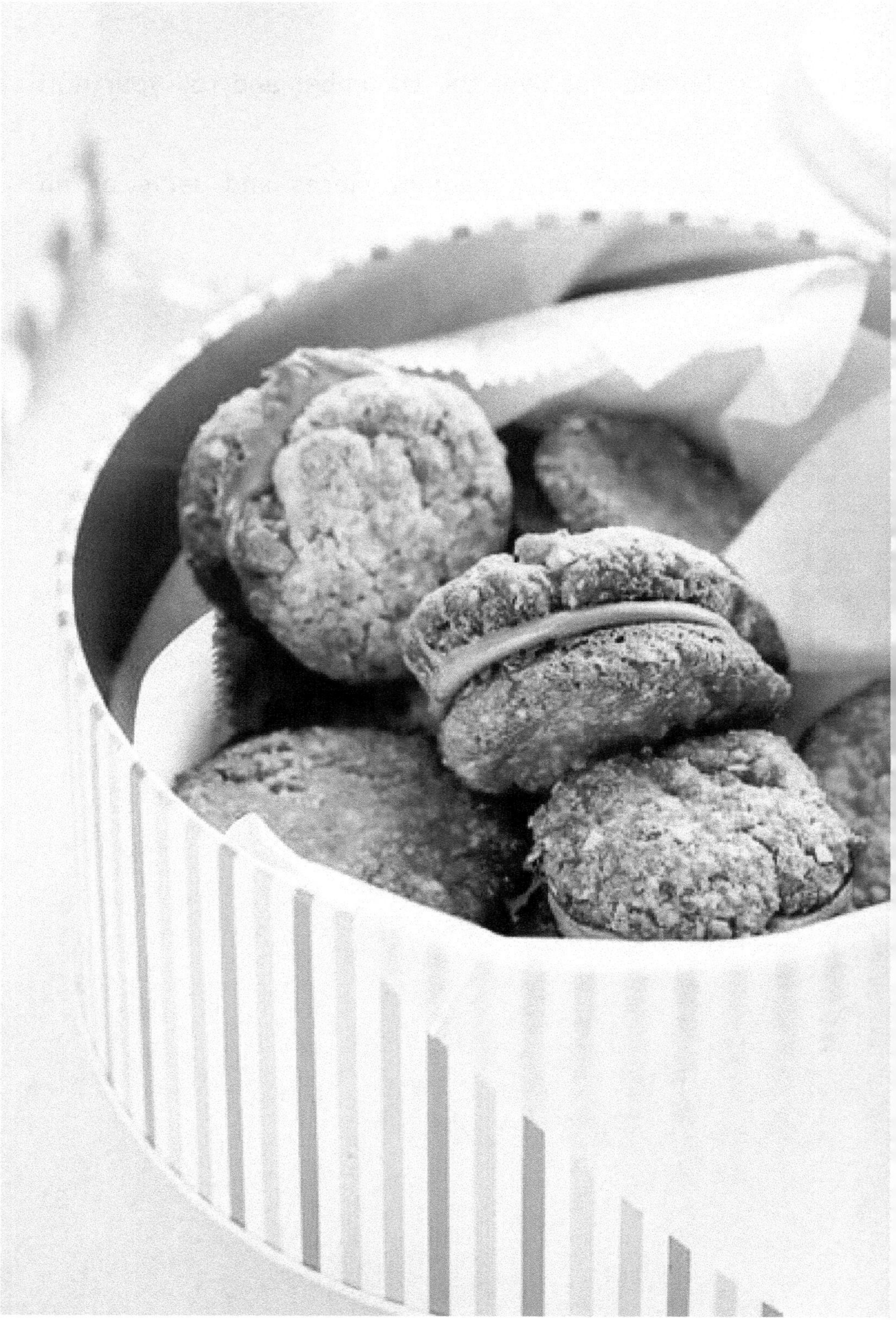

Mussels Appetizer

8 Servings

Preparation time: 20 minutes

Ingredients

- 3 Garlic cloves, minced
- 1 handful chopped Parsley
- 1 yellow Onion, chopped
- Salt and Black pepper to the taste
- 1 tablespoon Olive oil
- 2 pounds Mussels
- 2 ounces canned Crushed tomatoes
- 2 ounces canned Chopped tomatoes
- 2 tablespoons Chicken soup
- 1 teaspoon crushed Red pepper flakes

Directions

- Heat up a Dutch oven over medium-high heat with the oil, then add onion, stir and cook for 3 minutes.

- Add in the garlic, red pepper flakes, crushed and chopped tomatoes, then stir.
- Add the stock, salt, pepper, and the mussels, then toss, cook for a few minutes until the mussels open.
- Discard unopened mussels, then mix the opened mussels with the parsley.
- Toss the mix, divide into bowls and serve.

Ahi Tuna Appetizer

6 Servings

Preparation time: 17 minutes

Ingredients

- 1 Cauliflower head, florets separated and riced
- 2 tablespoons Green onions, chopped
- 1 Avocado, pitted, peeled and chopped
- 1 ahi tuna Steak
- 2 tablespoons Olive oil
- 1 Cucumber, grated

For the salad dressing

- 1 tablespoon Apple cider vinegar
- A pinch of Salt
- 1 tablespoon Sesame oil
- 2 tablespoons Coconut aminos

Directions

- Put some water in a pot, add a steamer basket inside, add cauliflower rice and bring to a boil over medium heat.
- Cover the pot, steam for a few minutes, then drain and divide into bowls.
- Heat up a pan with the coconut oil over medium-high heat and add the tuna.
- Cook for 1 minute on each side and divide into the bowls with the rice.
- Also, divide the green onions, cucumber and avocado among the bowls.
- In a separate small bowl, whisk together the sesame oil with the aminos, vinegar and a pinch of salt.
- Drizzle the dressing over the sushi bowls and serve as an appetizer.

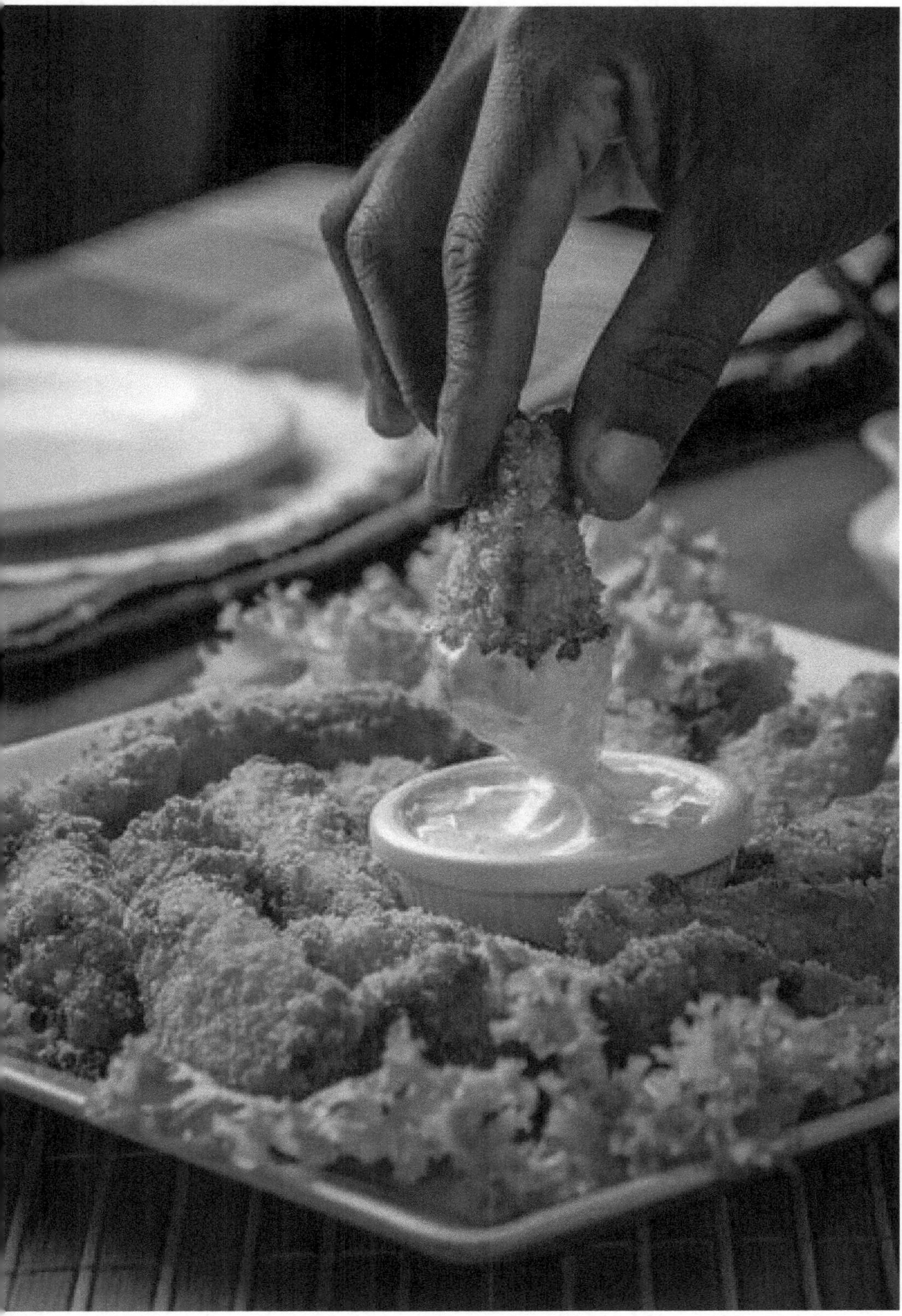

Chicken Bites

4 Servings

Preparation time: 20 minutes

Ingredients

- 2 Chicken breasts, cubed

- Salt and Black pepper to the taste

- ½ cup Coconut oil

- ½ cup Almond flour

- 1 Egg

- 2 tablespoons Garlic powder

Directions

- In a bowl, mix the garlic powder with the flour, salt and pepper and stir.
- In another bowl, beat the egg well.
- Dip the chicken breast pieces in the egg mix, then in flour mix.

- Heat up a pan with the oil over medium heat, then drop chicken pieces into the hot pan.
- Cook them for 5 minutes on each side, then divide into bowls and serve as a snack.

DINNER

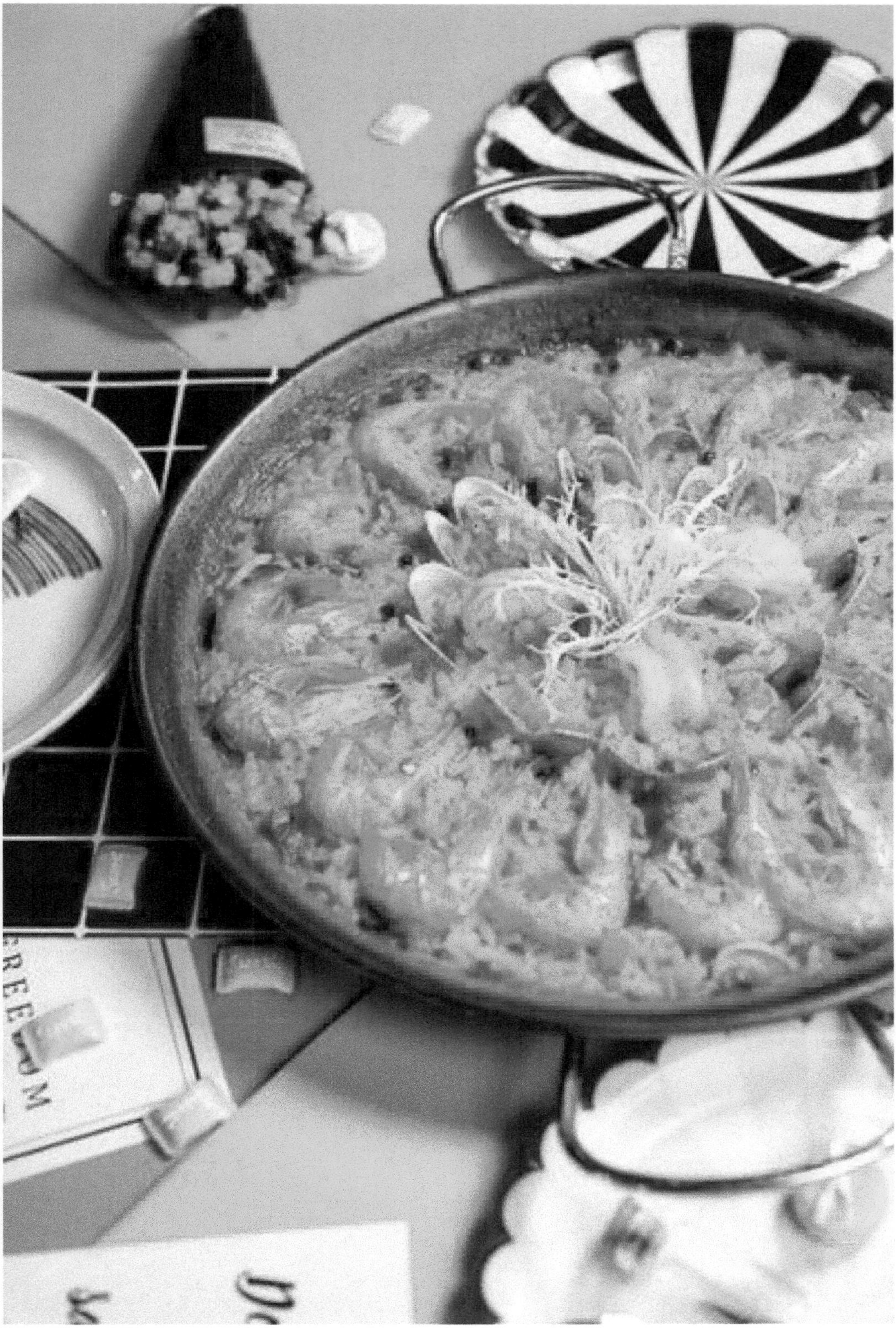

Curry Tilapia

3 Servings

Preparation Time: 25 minutes

Ingredients

- 14 oz Tilapia fillet, chopped
- 1 teaspoon Olive oil
- 1 teaspoon Curry powder
- ½ cup of Coconut milk

Directions

- Pour Olive oil into the pan and preheat it well.
- Add tilapia and cook it for 1 minute per side.
- Meanwhile, mix Coconut milk with curry powder.
- Pour the mixture over the fish and cook the meal for 10 minutes more.

Corn Bake

6 Servings

Preparation Time: 30 minutes

Ingredients

- 2 cups corn Kernels
- ¼ cup Coconut cream
- 4 oz Parmesan, grated
- 1 teaspoon dried basil

Directions

- In the mixing bowl, mix corn kernels with Coconut cream and dried basil.
- Add the mixture into the baking pan and top with Parmesan.
- Bake the corn bake at 360° for 20 minutes.

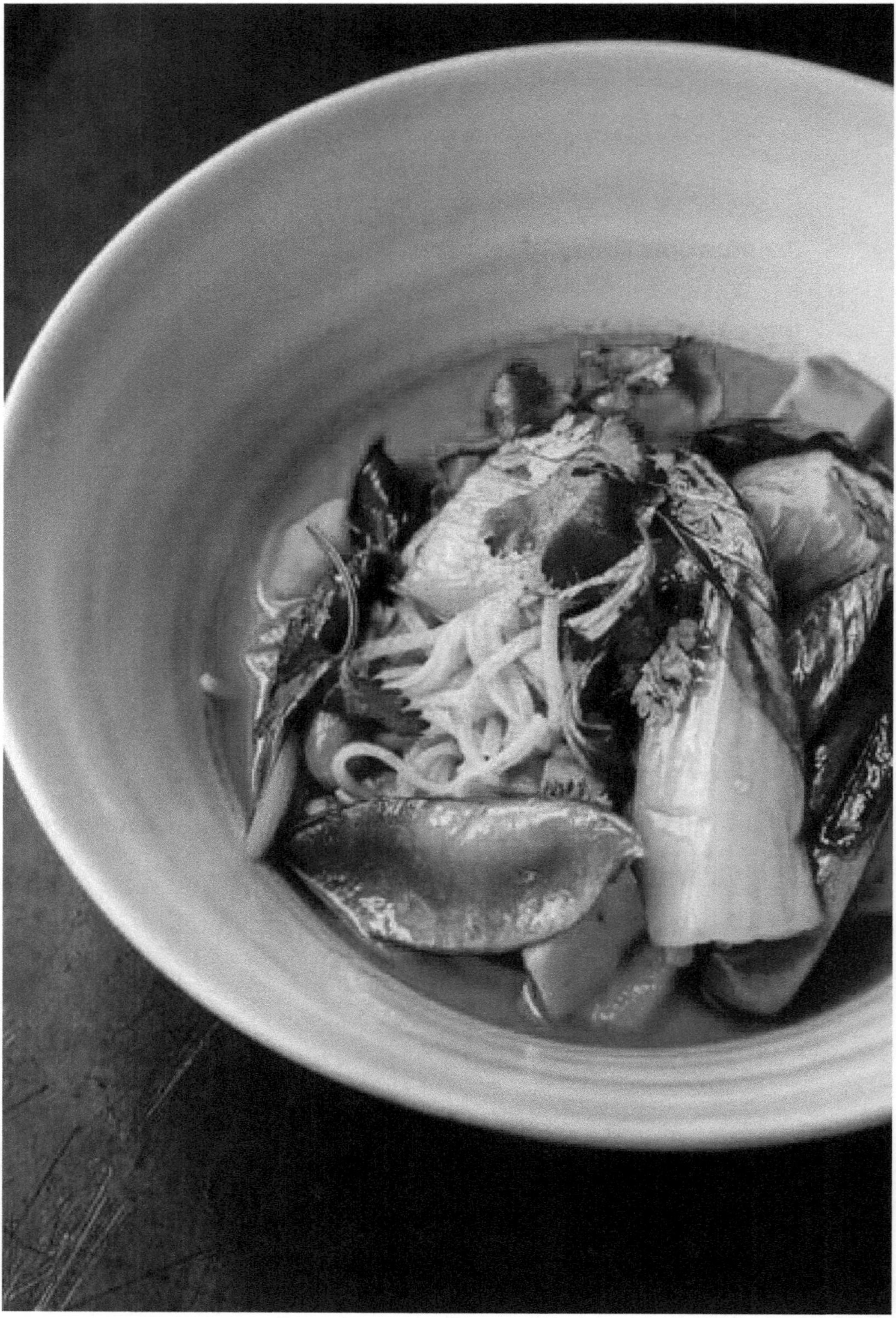

Baked Squash

5 Servings

Preparation Time: 35 minutes

Ingredients

- 4 Zucchinis, Halved
- 1 teaspoon dried Thyme
- ½ teaspoon Cayenne pepper
- 1 tablespoon Olive oil

Directions

- Sprinkle the zucchinis with Olive oil, dried thyme, and cayenne pepper.
- Add the zucchini halves in the tray and bake at 400° for 25 minutes.

Cinnamon Pumpkin Cubes

5 Servings

Preparation Time: 1 hour

Ingredients

- 1 teaspoon ground Cinnamon
- 1 tablespoon Olive oil
- 1 teaspoon dried Basil
- 2 cups Pumpkin, chopped

Directions

- Mix ground cinnamon with pumpkin, and dried basil.
- Then Add the pumpkin in the tray and sprinkle with Olive oil.
- Cook the pumpkin at 350° for 50 minutes in the oven.

Spicy Daikon Radish

6 Servings

Preparation Time: 10 minutes

Ingredients

- 1-pound daikon Radish, peeled, chopped
- 2 oz Chives, chopped
- 1/3 cup plain Yogurt
- 2 Cucumbers, chopped

Directions

- Add all ingredients into the mixing bowl.
- Carefully mix the meal and transfer it to the serving bowls.

Honey Duck Fillet

6 Servings

Preparation Time: 25 minutes

Ingredients

- 1-pound duck fillet, chopped
- 1 tablespoon raw honey
- 1 teaspoon ground turmeric
- ½ teaspoon dried mint
- 1 tablespoon Olive oil

Directions

- Mix duck fillet with dried mint and ground turmeric.
- Then preheat the Olive oil and add the duck pieces inside.
- Roast them for 10 minutes. Stir the meat from time to time.
- After this, add honey and carefully mix the meal.
- Close the lid and cook it for 5 minutes more.

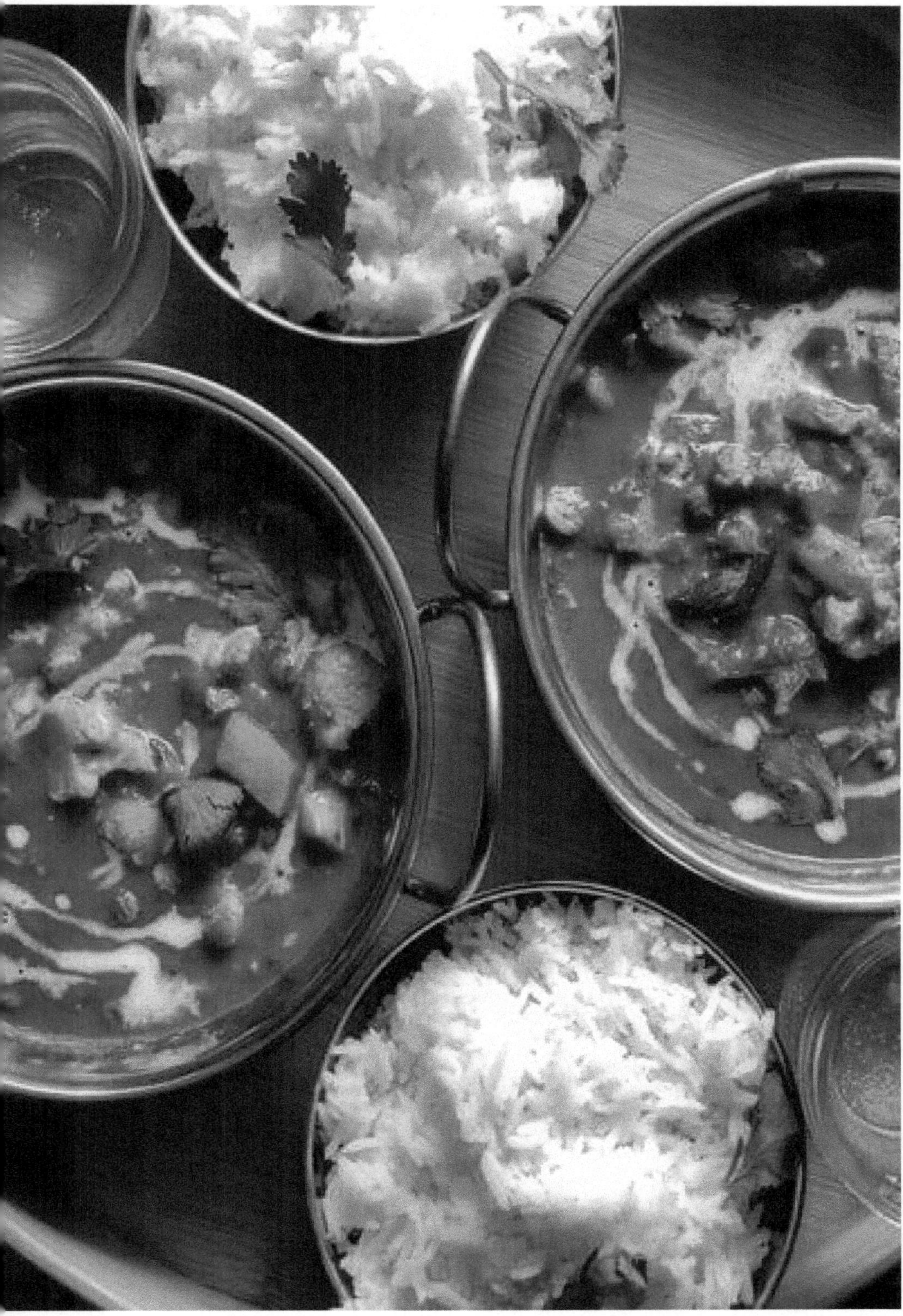

Sweet Chicken Bake

6 Servings

Preparation Time: 40 minutes

Ingredients

- 1-pound Chicken fillet, chopped
- 1 cup peaches, chopped
- ½ cup of Water
- 1 teaspoon ground nutmeg
- 1 teaspoon ground clove
- ½ lemon, chopped

Directions

- Mix the Chicken fillet with ground nutmeg and ground clove.
- Add the Chicken to the baking pan.
- Add water, lemon, and peaches.
- Close the lid and cook the meal in the oven at 365° for 30 minutes.

Tomato Chicken

6 Servings

Preparation Time: 35 minutes

Ingredients

- 1 onion, diced
- 2 cups Tomatoes, chopped
- 1 chili pepper, chopped
- 1 Garlic clove, chopped
- 1 tablespoon Olive oil
- 1-pound Chicken fillet, chopped

Directions

- Add all ingredients in the saucepan and carefully mix.
- Close the lid and cook the Chicken for 25 minutes on medium heat.
- Stir the Chicken from time to time to avoid burning.

SOUPS

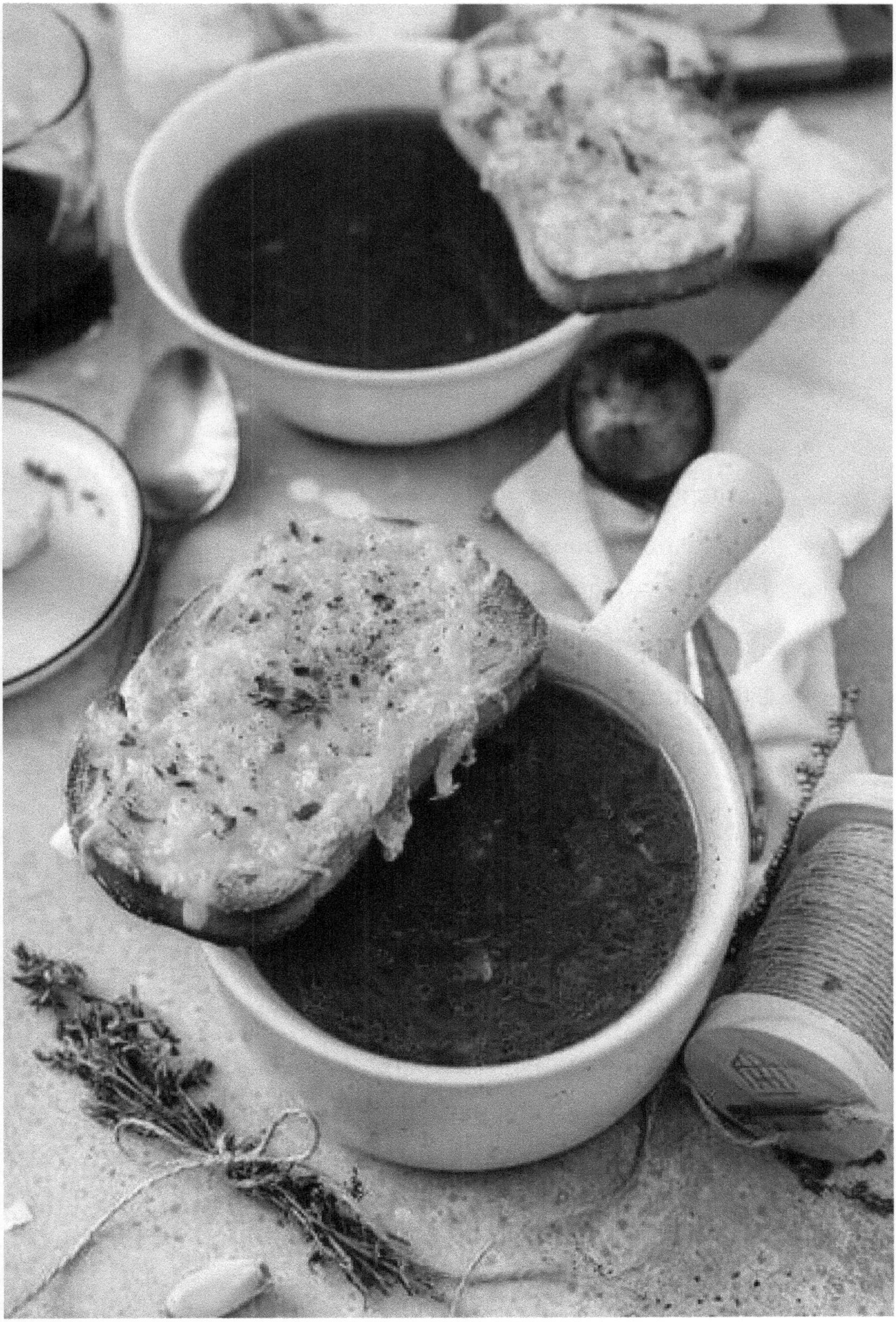

Ginger Cauliflower Soup

6 Servings

Preparation Time: 45 minutes

Ingredients

- 2 carrots peeled and grated.
- 1 pound cauliflower, chopped.
- 1 teaspoon minced. garlic
- 1 tablespoon olive oil
- 1 teaspoon chili powder
- 4 cups of water
- 1 teaspoon ginger, grated.
- Half cup fresh cilantro, chopped.

Directions

- Pour olive oil in the saucepan.
- Add minced. Garlic, ginger, and chili powder.
- Mix the mixture and cook it for 2 minutes.
- Then add all remaining ingredients and carefully mix the soup with the help of the spoon.
- Cook it for 23 minutes.

Tomato Soup

6 Servings

Preparation Time: 50 minutes

Ingredients

- 4 cups tomatoes, chopped.
- 2 cups of water
- Half cup fresh spinach, chopped.
- 1 teaspoon garlic, diced.
- 1 teaspoon ground paprika
- 1 teaspoon cayenne pepper
- 1 cup broccoli, chopped.

Directions

- Put all ingredients in the saucepan and close the lid.
- Simmer the soup for 20 minutes on medium heat.
- Blend the soup with the help of the immersion blender.
- Bring the cream soup to a boil and cook for 5 minutes more.

Broccoli Soup

6 Servings

Preparation Time: 45 minutes

Ingredients

- 1 yellow onion, chopped.
- 1 carrot, chopped.
- 2 cups broccoli, hopped.
- 1 tablespoon olive oil
- 5 cups of water
- 1 cup tomatoes, chopped.
- 1 teaspoon chili powder

Directions

- Pour olive oil in the saucepan.
- Add onion and carrot. Roast the vegetables for 5 minutes on medium heat.
- Then add broccoli, water, tomatoes, and chili powder.
- Close the lid and cook the soup on medium heat for 30 minutes.

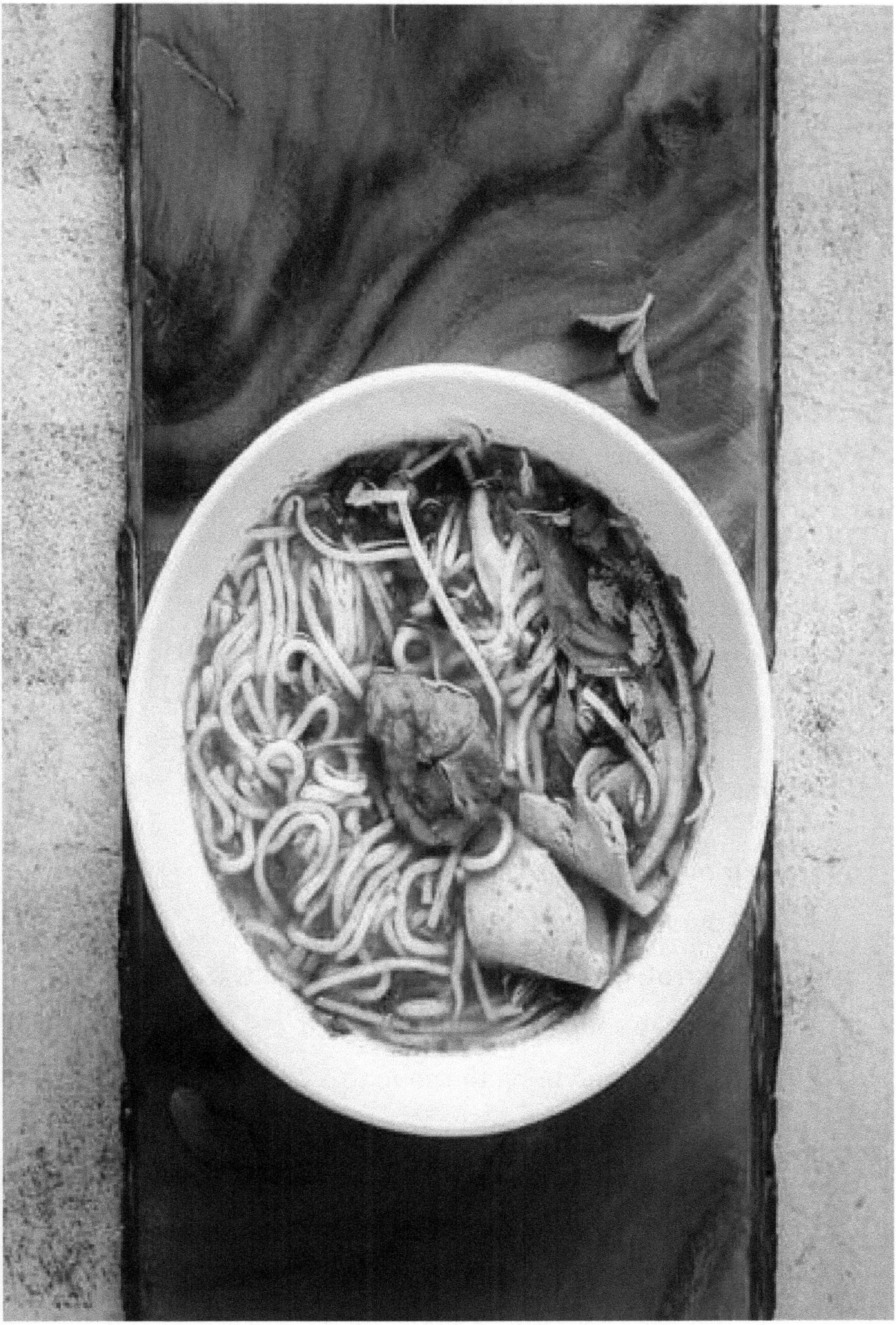

Spinach Soup

6 Servings

Preparation Time: 40 minutes

Ingredients

- 1 cup carrot, grated.
- 2 cups spinach, chopped.
- 1 onion, diced.
- 1 tablespoon olive oil
- 1 teaspoon garlic powder
- 1 teaspoon dried dill
- 5 cups of water

Directions

- Pour olive oil in the saucepan.
- Add onion and roast it until light brown.
- Add carrot, garlic powder, dried dill, and water.
- Simmer the soup for 10 minutes.
- Add spinach and bring the soup to a boil.

Yellow Soup

6 Servings

Preparation Time: 45 minutes

Ingredients

- 2 cups carrot, chopped.
- 1 cup pumpkin, chopped.
- 1 teaspoon ground cinnamon
- 1 tablespoon lemon juice
- 1 teaspoon lemon zest, grated.
- 6 cups of water

Directions

- Put all ingredients in the saucepan and close the lid.
- Cook the soup on medium heat for 25 minutes or until all ingredients are soft.

Onion Cream Soup

6 Servings

Preparation Time: 40 minutes

Ingredients

- 2 cups onions, chopped.
- 5 cups of water
- 1 cup sweet pepper, chopped.
- 2 tbsps olive oil
- 1 tablespoon dried dill
- 1 teaspoon ground paprika
- 2 ounces Parmesan, grated.

Directions

- Mix olive oil with onions in the saucepan and roast the mixture for 5 minutes.
- Then add water, sweet pepper, dried dill, and ground paprika.
- Close the lid and cook the soup for 15 minutes more.

- Then blend it with the help of the immersion blender.
- Top the soup with Parmesan.

Green Peas Soup

8 Servings

Preparation Time: 55 minutes

Ingredients

- 1 onion, chopped.
- 1-pound green peas
- 1 carrot, grated.
- 6 cups of water
- 1 tablespoon dried sage
- 1 teaspoon cayenne pepper
- 2 tbsps olive oil

Directions

- Pour olive oil in the saucepan. Add carrot and roast it for 5 minutes.
- Then add onion, green peas, sage, and cayenne pepper.
- Close the lid and simmer the soup on low heat for 30 minutes.

Red Soup

8 Servings

Preparation Time: 50 minutes

Ingredients

- 2 cups cabbage, shredded.
- 2 cups tomatoes, chopped.
- 4 ounces leek, chopped.
- 6 cups of water
- 1 cup tomato juice

Directions

- Pour water in the saucepan. Add tomatoes and bring the mixture to a boil.
- Then blend the mixture until smooth.
- Add cabbage, leek, and tomato juice.
- Simmer the soup for 20 minutes on low heat.

DESSERTS

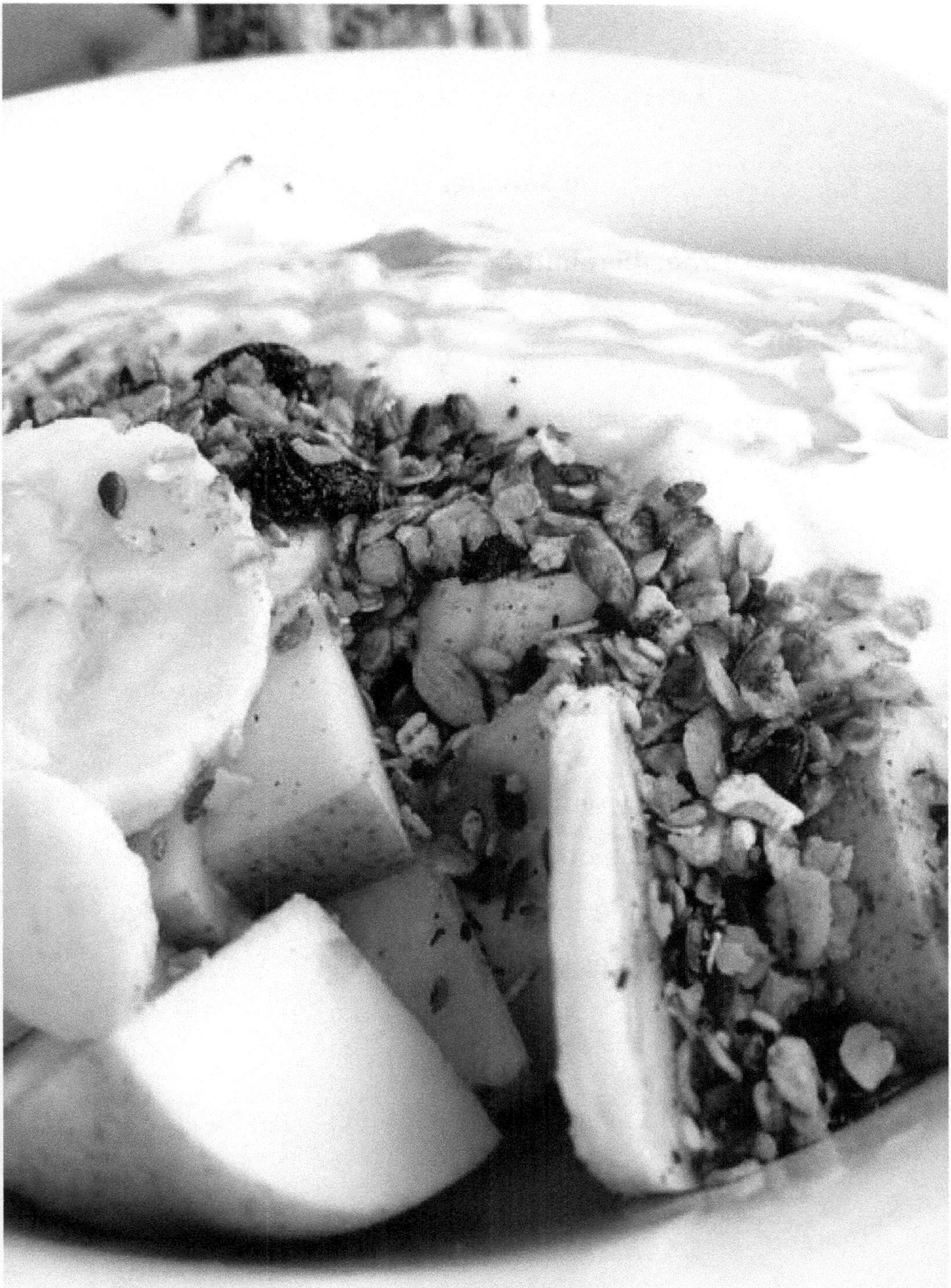

Lemon Coconut Cream

6 Servings

Preparation Time: 45 minutes

Ingredients

- 2 cups coconut cream
- Juice of 1 lemon
- Zest of 1 lemon, grated.
- 1 teaspoon vanilla extract
- 2 tbsps chicory root powder

Directions

- In a bowl, combine the cream with the lemon juice and the other ingredients.
- Whisk, divide into bowls and keep in the fridge for 30 minutes before serving.

Honey Berry Curd

6 Servings

Preparation Time: 30 minutes

Ingredients

- 2 cups blackberries
- Quarter cup lime juice
- 2 tbsps honey
- 2 teaspoons lime zest, grated.
- 4 tbsps coconut oil, melted.
- 3 egg yolks, whisked.

Directions

- Heat up a small pan over medium heat, add the berries and lime juice.
- Mix, bring to a simmer, cook for 5 minutes, strain this into a heatproof bowl and mash a bit.
- Put some water into a pan, bring to a simmer over medium heat, and add the bowl with the berries on top.

- Add the rest of the ingredients, mix well, cook for 5 minutes more, divide into small cups, and serve cold.

Coconut Avocado Pie

8 Servings

Preparation Time: 1 hour and 20 minutes

Ingredients

- 2 cups coconut flour
- 6 tbsps coconut butter
- 5 tbsps water
- For the filling:
- 2 avocados, peeled, pitted. And cubed.
- 3 tbsps chicory root powder
- 3 tbsps almond flour
- Half teaspoon vanilla extract
- 2 eggs, whisked.
- 1 tablespoon coconut oil, melted.
- 2 tbsps coconut milk

Directions

- In a bowl, mix the coconut flour with the coconut butter and the water, mix until you obtain a firm dough.

- Transfer the dough to a floured working surface, knead it, shape a flattened disk, wrap in plastic, keep in the fridge for 30 minutes, roll a circle and arrange in a pie pan.
- In a bowl, mix the avocados with the chicory root powder and the other ingredients for the filling.
- Mix well, pour into the pie pan, introduce in the oven at 370 degrees F, and bake for 40 minutes, cut, and serve.

Coconut Carrot Cake

8 Servings

Preparation Time: 55 minutes

Ingredients

- 2 cups coconut milk
- Half cup coconut oil, melted.
- Chicory root powder to the taste
- 4 eggs, whisked.
- 2 carrots, grated.
- 2 teaspoons vanilla extract
- 2 cups almond flour
- 1 teaspoon baking soda

Directions

- In a bowl, combine the milk with coconut oil and the other ingredients.
- Mix well, pour into a cake pan, bake in the oven at 350 degrees F for 35 minutes, slice, divide between plates and serve.

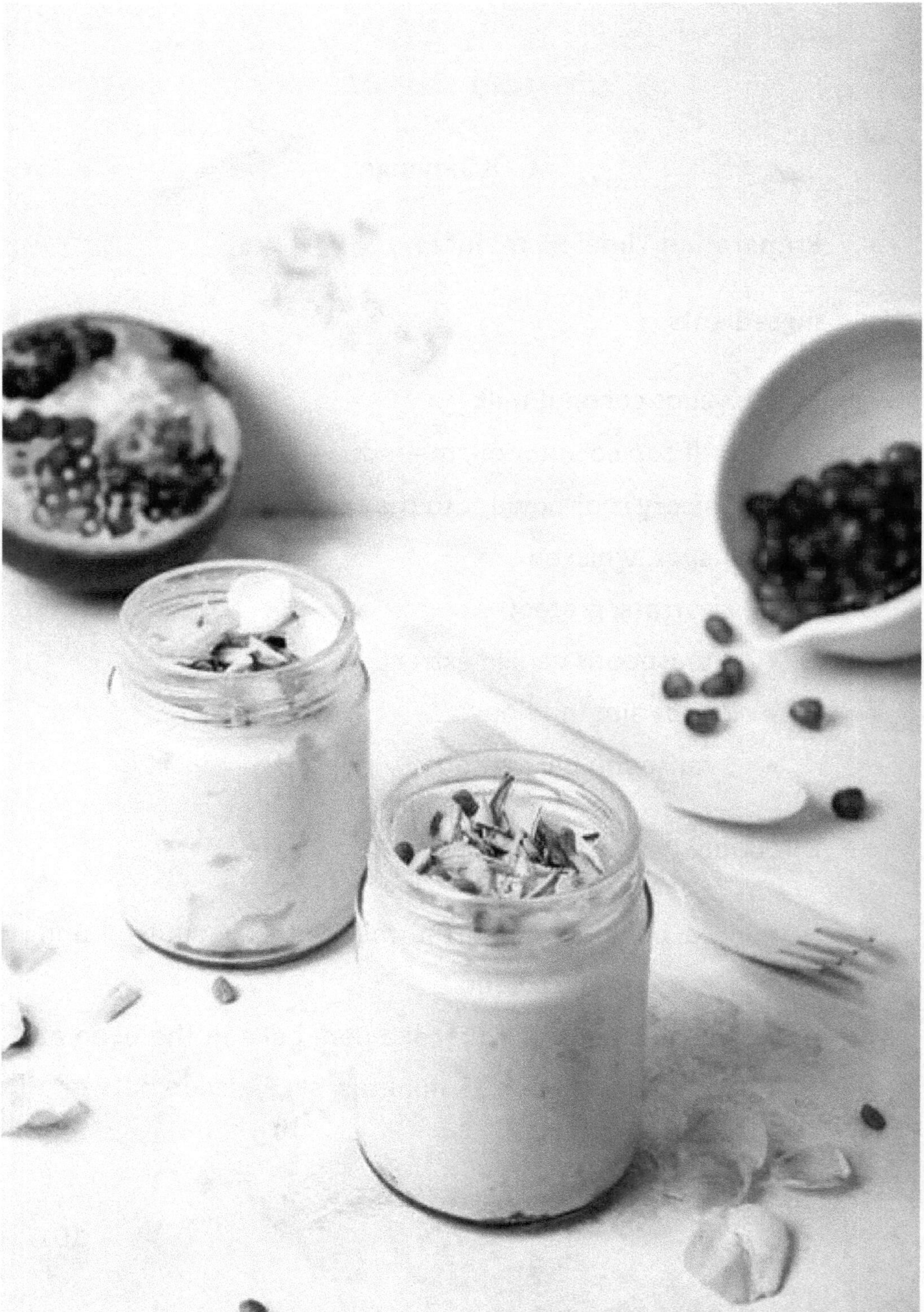

Quinoa Pudding

6 Servings

Preparation Time: 35 minutes

Ingredients

- 1 cup quinoa
- 2 cups almond milk
- 3 tbsps coconut butter
- Quarter cup almonds, chopped.
- 1 tablespoon chicory root powder
- Half cup pomegranate seeds.

Directions

- In a pot, combine the quinoa with the almond milk and the other ingredients.
- Bring to a simmer and cook over medium heat for 20 minutes.
- Divide into bowls and serve cold.

Green Tea Pudding

6 Servings

Preparation Time: 35 minutes

Ingredients

- 3 cups almond milk
- Half cup coconut cream
- 2 tbsps green tea powder
- 1 teaspoon vanilla extract
- 3 tbsps chicory root powder

Directions

- In a pot, combine the almond milk with the cream and the other ingredients.
- Whisk, bring to a simmer and cook over medium heat for 15 minutes.
- Divide the mix into bowls and serve.

Blackberry Cream

6 Servings

Preparation Time: 10 minutes

Ingredients

- 1 cup blackberries
- 1 cup pineapple peeled and cubed.
- 1 tablespoon coconut oil, melted.
- ¾ cup coconut cream
- 2 tbsps maple syrup

Directions

- In your blender, combine the berries with the pineapple and the other ingredients.
- Pulse well, divide into bowls and serve cold.

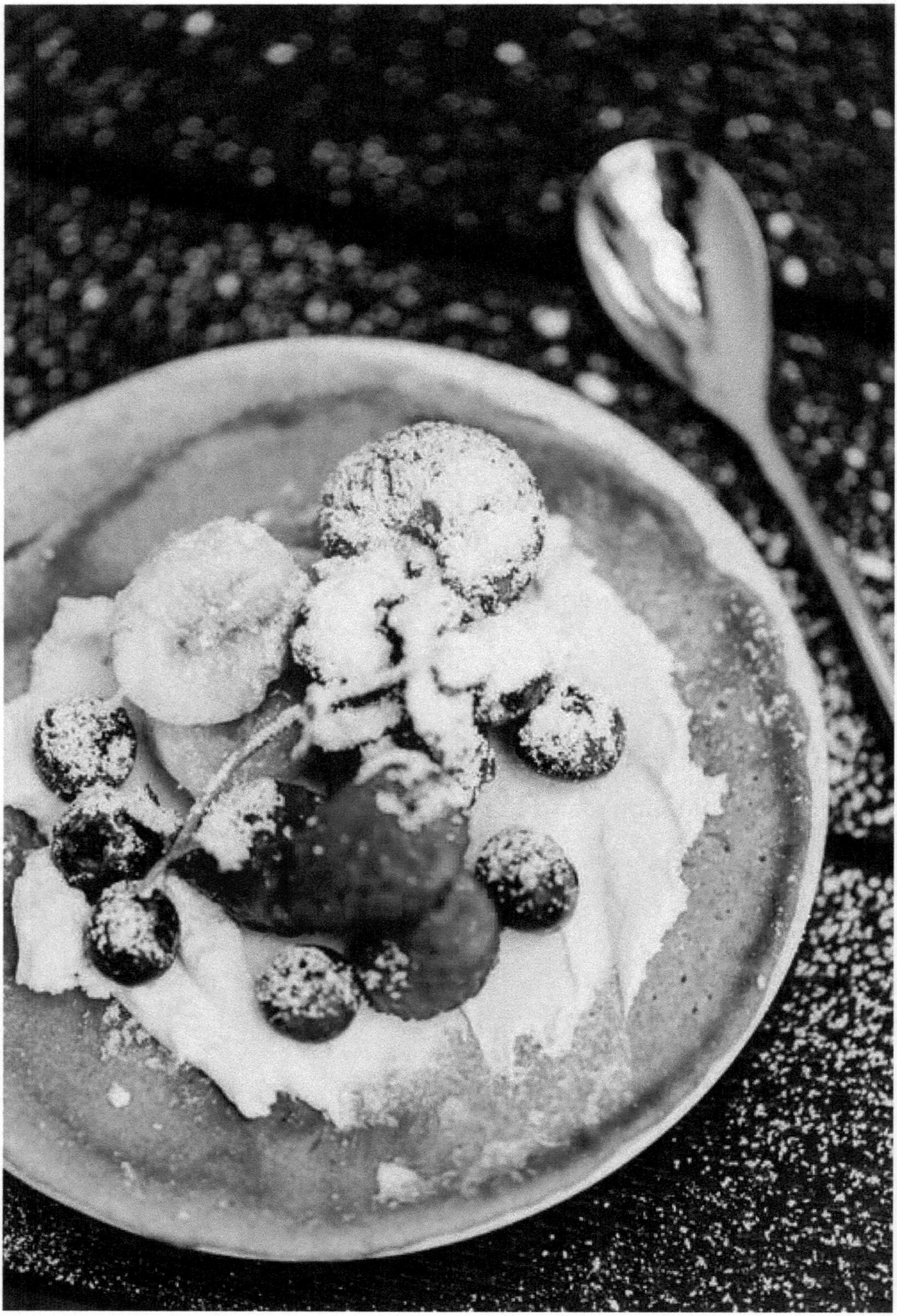

Strawberries Pudding

6 Servings

Preparation Time: 45 minutes

Ingredients

- 2 cups almond milk
- 1 cup black rice
- Half cup strawberries
- 2 tbsps chicory root powder
- 1 teaspoon cinnamon powder

Directions

- Heat up a pan with the milk over medium heat; add the rice and the other ingredients.
- Cook for 25 minutes, mixing often, divide into bowls and serve cold.

Coconut Grapes Bowls

6 Servings

Preparation Time: 45 minutes

Ingredients

- 2 cups coconut milk
- Half cup coconut cream
- Half cup black tea
- 1 teaspoon vanilla extract
- 1 cup grapes cut in halves.
- 1 tablespoon chicory root powder
- 1 tablespoon maple syrup

Directions

- Heat up a pan with the coconut milk over medium heat; add the cream, the grapes, and the other ingredients.
- Bring to a simmer and cook over medium heat for 25 minutes.
- Divide into bowls and serve cold.